WARD LO

FAMILY HEALTH G

DIABETES

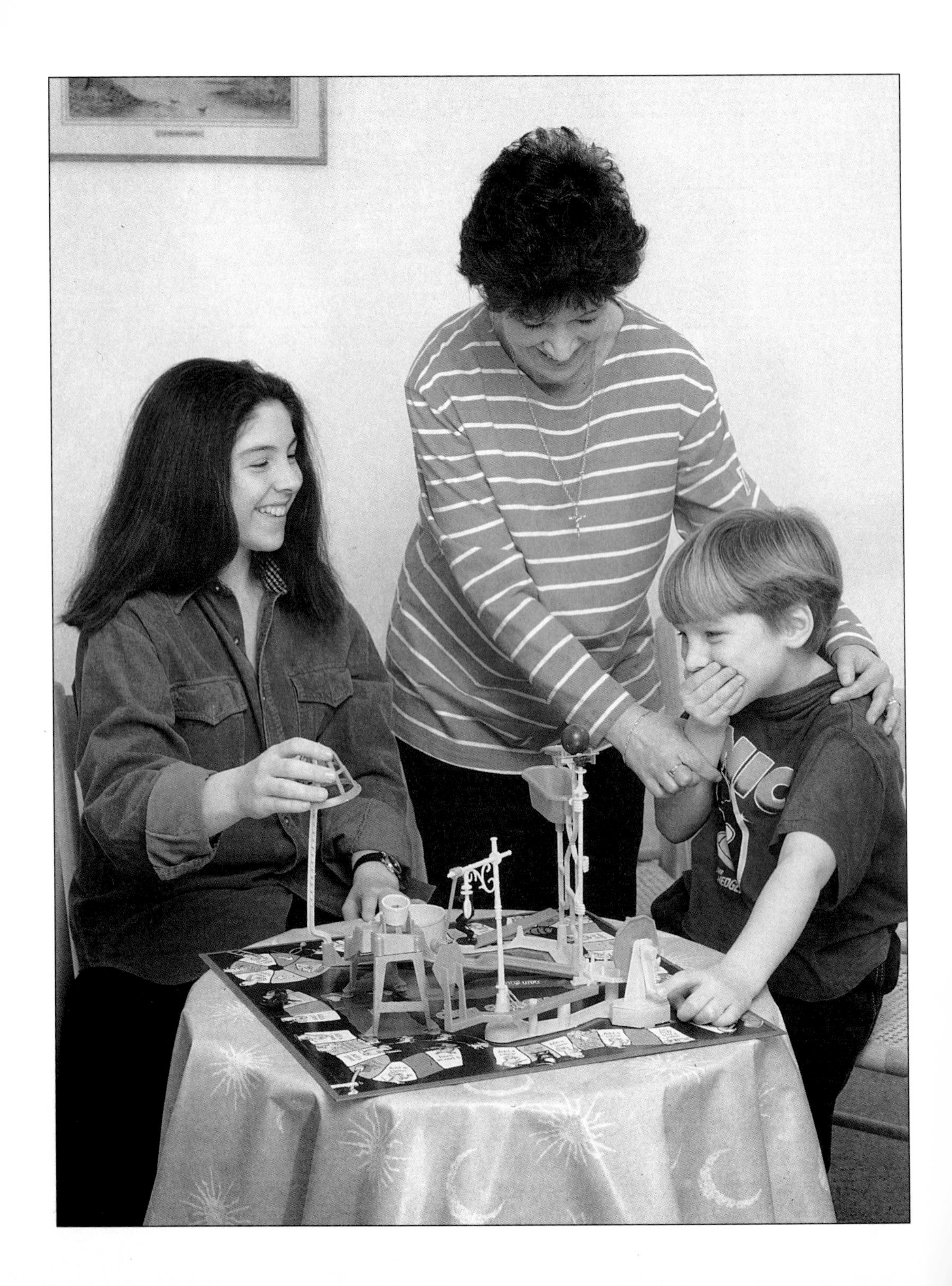

WARD LOCK

FAMILY HEALTH GUIDE

DIABETES

CHRIS McLAUGHLIN

WITH THE HELP OF
THE BRITISH DIABETIC ASSOCIATION

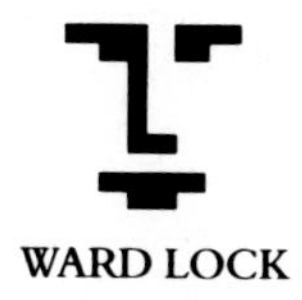

WARD LOCK

Chris McLaughlin
Chris McLaughlin is a freelance writer who specializes in health matters. She writes regular health features for a wide range of national newspapers, women's and health magazines in the UK. She is the co-owner of a writing and editing agency and has written several books.

A WARD LOCK BOOK

First published in the UK 1994
by Ward Lock
Villiers House
41/47 Strand
London
WC2N 5JE

A Cassell Imprint

Designed and produced
by SP Creative Design
147 Kings Road, Bury St Edmunds, Suffolk, England

Editor: Heather Thomas
Art director: Al Rockall
Designer: Rolando Ugolini
Illustrations: Rolando Ugolini

Distributed in the United States
by Sterling Publishing Co., Inc.
387 Park Avenue South, New York, NY 10016-8810

Distributed in Australia
by Capricorn Link(Australia) Pty Ltd
2/13 Carrington Road, Castle Hill, NSW 2154

A British Library Cataloguing in Publication Data block for this book may be obtained from the British Library.

ISBN 0 7063 7258 1

Printed and bound in Spain

Acknowledgements
The publishers would like to extend special thanks to the British Diabetic Association for their invaluable help in producing this book.
Cover photograph: Image Bank/Juan Alvarez (posed by a model)
British Diabetic Association: photos on pages 2, 10, 12, 13, 15, 20, 24, 26, 33, 34, 36, 42, 43, 44, 45, 47, 48, 51, 52, 54, 56, 57, 58, 61, 63, 66, 67, 68, 71, 73, 74, 75, 76
Bayer Diagnostics: photos on pages 16, 31, 39

Contents

Introduction

The discovery that you or someone close to you is suffering from diabetes is almost always a shock, and raises all kinds of questions about the effects it will have on the lives of the sufferer and those closest to him or her. It inevitably takes time for the implications to sink in. Many people worry that their lives will be very restricted in future or even that they will become invalids. In fact, there is no reason why a person with diabetes shouldn't live a perfectly normal life, even though they will have to make certain adjustments, and probably need some form of medical treatment to keep their illness under control.

First, let's get the bad news out of the way: at the moment, there is no cure for the condition because the basic fault which is responsible for causing the symptoms cannot be corrected. The good news is that, for the majority of people, treatment and self-help can keep the condition under control and minimize the risk of complications developing. Many people with diabetes develop an excellent understanding of their illness, which helps them to work with the experts to maintain their well-being.

Before looking at what help is available, we need to understand what goes wrong when diabetes develops.

Chapter one

What is diabetes?

The key to the problem of diabetes is in its proper medical name – diabetes mellitus – which actually means something like 'a fountain of sugar'. The name derives from the fact that people with this condition produce lots of very sweet urine because their bodies have lost the ability to control the level of sugar (or glucose) in their bloodstream. This loss may be total, as in people who have so-called Type I (insulin dependent, or IDDM)) or partial as in people who have Type II (non-insulin dependent, or NIDDMM).

In a healthy person, the digestive system converts starchy foods in our diet into glucose, and this, together with sugar from sweet foods is transported via the bloodstream into all the cells in our body. Glucose is the energy source which fuels all the activities of our body cells, but it needs the action of a hormone called insulin to get it into the cells. Any excess glucose which isn't required for the time being is stored away as glycogen in the liver, or as fat. If the level of glucose in our blood drops, perhaps because we haven't eaten enough or have been doing strenuous exercise and burned it all up, more glucose is released for conversion from the breakdown of body stores of fat and protein.

Normally, insulin levels rise and fall as required to keep the level of blood glucose more or less constant. The insulin is actually a hormone which comes from an organ called the pancreas, situated just behind the stomach and below the liver. In people with diabetes, this system of energy production and control breaks down, either because the pancreas simply stops producing insulin altogether (as in IDDM),or produces insufficient or ineffective insulin (as in NIDDMM).

When the insulin supply fails or is not effective at performing its task of conversion, the glucose cannot enter the cells where it is needed, and the level of glucose in the blood just goes on rising. The cells don't get their proper supply of energy, so the body tries to correct this. The liver releases extra quantities of glucose, and body tissue is broken down and converted into yet more glucose. Eventually, the bloodstream becomes so overloaded that it can't hold any more, and the excess is excreted in the urine via the kidneys.

If nothing is done to interrupt this process, a person who is producing no insulin at all will simply go on breaking down fats. One of the byproducts of the breakdown is acids called ketones which are released into the bloodstream and then into the urine. Eventually their presence could lead to a serious condition called diabetic keto-acidosis, or diabetic coma.

What is diabetes?

Which type of diabetes?

Most people think of a person with diabetes as someone who needs to give themselves regular injections of insulin to survive. In fact, the type of diabetes which is treated in this way – and called, logically enough, insulin dependent diabetes (or IDDM) – is not the most common. Because it normally starts before the age of 40, it is also sometimes referred to as 'childhood' or 'juvenile' diabetes. Doctors and other experts will often refer to it as Type I.

The symptoms can come on fairly quickly – in days or weeks rather than months – and are caused by the lack of insulin available. The majority of people with Type I produce no insulin at all, or, at best, minimal amounts, and so will have to take it artificially for the rest of their lives.

No one knows for sure why it happens, although it's possible that an as-yet unidentified virus may be responsible for damaging the cells in the pancreas. Another possibility is that the body's immune system, which is designed to attack and destroy invaders like bacteria and viruses, turns instead on itself. This kind of thing is known to happen in some other illnesses such as rheumatoid arthritis, but no one is as yet sure why, nor is it certain whether it is a factor in diabetes. Very occasionally, the

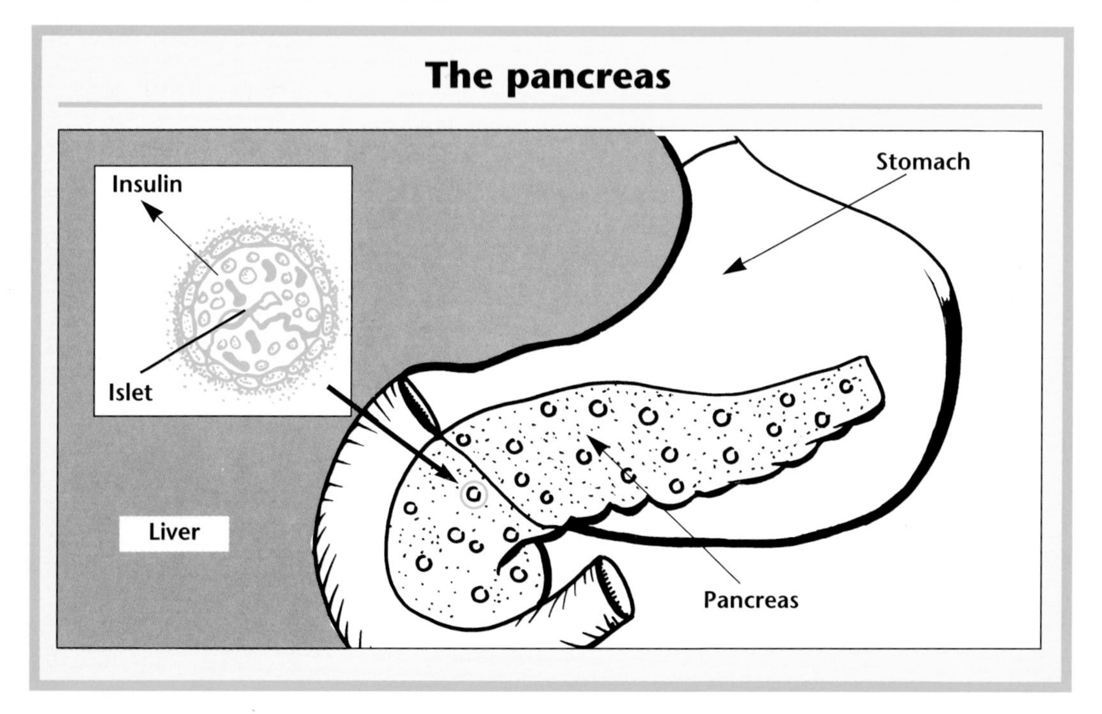

cause may be some kind of disease of the pancreas or, even less common, certain kinds of hormone imbalance. In most cases, however, the specific cause isn't known.

The other, more common, type of diabetes comes on much more slowly as the insulin-producing cells gradually become less efficient or as the insulin they produce works less effectively. Type II, or, as it used to be called, 'maturity onset diabetes', is thought to account for some 90 per cent of all cases of diabetes in this country. Because sufferers usually still produce some insulin, and most of them don't require injections, it is also known as non-insulin dependent diabetes (or NIDDMM).

No one knows why some people develop this type of diabetes in later life, although those who are overweight seem to be more vulnerable. The symptoms can be caused in one of two ways:

- Either the supply of insulin from the pancreas slows down so that there isn't enough to convert all the blood glucose into energy or fat.
- Or the person develops what's known as 'insulin resistance'. What this means is that although the body is still churning out the hormone, it no longer produces the desired effect because the person has somehow become less sensitive to it.

Either way, the result is the same. There will be too much glucose in the bloodstream, and some of the excess will spill over to make the urine sweet. The onset is much slower than with Type I, and it may be years before the symptoms are noticeable enough to get the sufferer to the doctor's.

The main symptoms of diabetes are listed below. The rate at which they occur and the degree of their severity varies from one individual to another. However, once diabetes has been diagnosed and is treated, these symptoms can be relieved quickly.

Symptoms of IDDM

- Needing to pass urine very frequently and in large quantities.
- Severe thirst and a dry mouth.
- Extreme tiredness and fatigue.
- Sudden and dramatic loss of weight.
- Itching around the genital organs.
- Blurred vision.

If allowed to go untreated, they may eventually result in dehydration, vomiting and diabetic coma.

Symptoms of NIDDMM

- Feeling permanently tired for no obvious reason.
- Needing to drink more fluid than is usual.
- Having to pass urine frequently and in large quantities.
- Frquent skin problems, such as boils and itching in the genital area.
- Blurred vision.
- Pain or tingling sensations in the fingers and legs.

Note that the onset of these symptoms is more gradual and less sudden than with IDDM, and they are usually less severe. Diabetic coma does not occur.

What is diabetes?

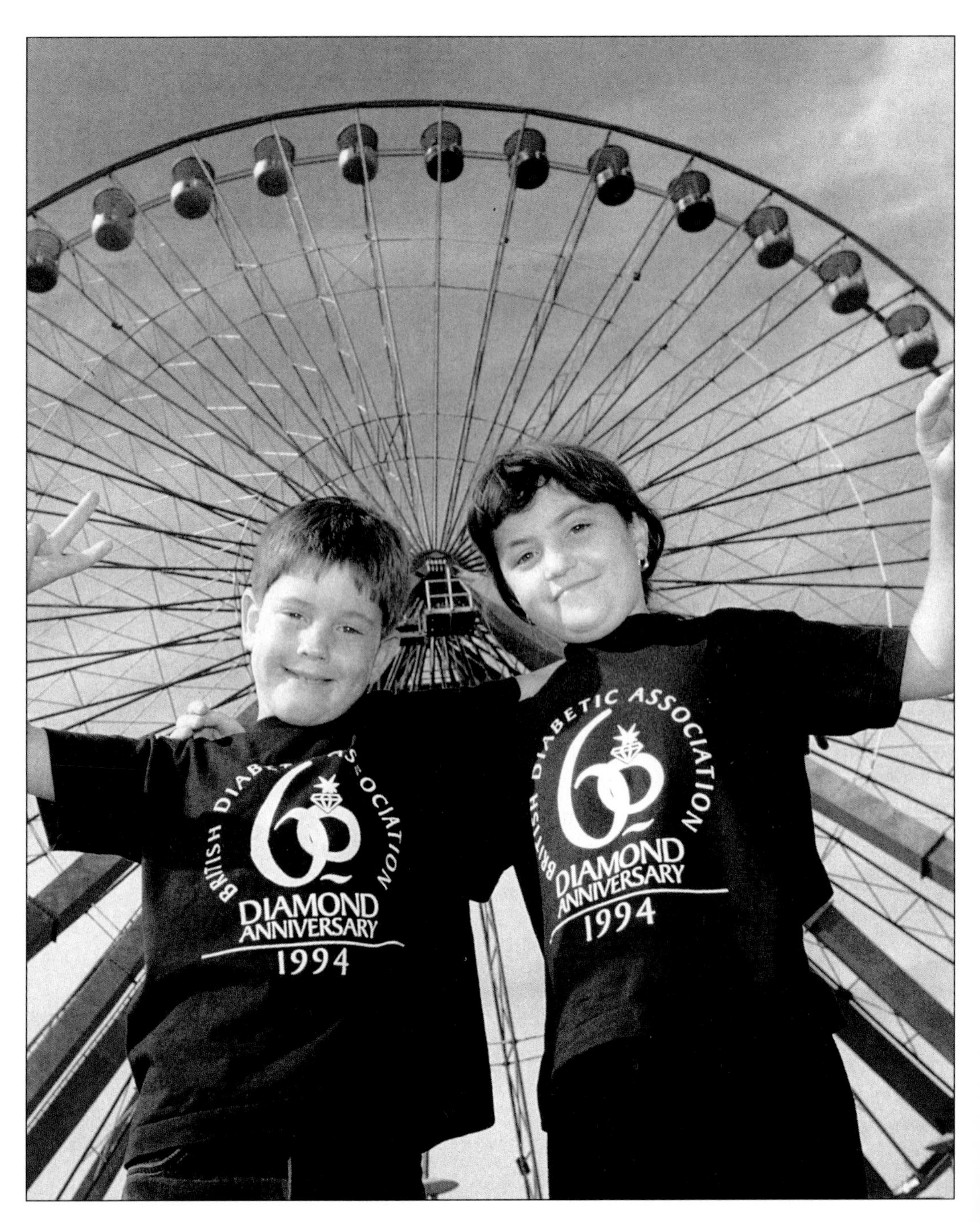

Who develops diabetes?

The simple answer is an awful lot of people. Estimates suggest that some one to two per cent of the population in the UK have diabetes, although many of them may not know it. This could mean that there are as many as one million sufferers, of whom around 18,000 are young people under 20. It's rare among babies, but often comes on in young people at around 12, when their bodies are going through a period of important hormonal changes. Boys and girls are affected in about equal numbers.

Among older people, however, the picture is slightly different, with more women than men having the condition. One of the reasons that the number of people with diabetes is currently growing – and expected to carry on doing so – is that non-insulin dependent diabetes usually affects middle-aged and older people, and the proportion of people in the population in this age group is increasing.

In both kinds of diabetes there seems to be some family link; if a close relative has diabetes, you are more likely to be affected. However, this link is stronger where non-insulin dependent diabetes is concerned. Some people have suggested that this may be partly because it is also more common in overweight or obese people, and this tendency may run in families too.

Nevertheless, it is important to remember that a lot of people who carry a genetic tendency to develop diabetes never actually do so. For example, if one of a pair of identical twins develops insulin dependent diabetes, the chances of the other one doing so are only 50:50. In any case, the majority of young people who have the condition do not turn out to have a parent or other close relative who also has the disease.

So while it is clear that there is some inherited tendency to develop diabetes, especially the non-insulin dependent sort, it is also plain that there must be some other factor at work which determines who gets it and who doesn't. Carrying excess weight seems to play some part in non-insulin dependent diabetes, while a virus or some other infection is probably responsible for triggering the condition in those who are genetically predisposed to suffering from the insulin dependent kind.

How diabetes is diagnosed

If you experience any or all of the symptoms listed above, you should see your doctor without delay. Insulin dependent diabetes is fatal if untreated, and while the consequences of untreated non-insulin dependent diabetes are less dramatic, they can still be serious. In particular, research has shown that many people already had signs of the particular kind

What is diabetes?

of eye damage it can cause (diabetic retinopathy or scarring of the retina, see page 60) by the time their condition was diagnosed. Many of these people also had raised blood pressure, and doctors believe that the delay in starting treatment could make them more prone to other medical complications.

Your doctor will ask you about your symptoms, and take down details of your medical history if he does not already know you and your family well. Suspected diabetes may be confirmed by urine and blood tests. These will often have to be sent off to the laboratory for analysis, and you will be asked to come back for the results in a few days.

The urine sample will be tested for the presence of glucose and ketones – the waste products produced when fat is broken down. A drop of blood, taken by pricking your finger or earlobe, is mixed with a chemical reagent on a special strip. Many doctors have the necessary equipment to do this in the surgery. The strip is simply placed in a gadget called a blood glucose meter, and it displays your blood glucose level.

Higher than normal readings from either or both of these tests, together with your symptoms, make it likely that you have diabetes, and your doctor may be able to confirm it definitely once he has the test

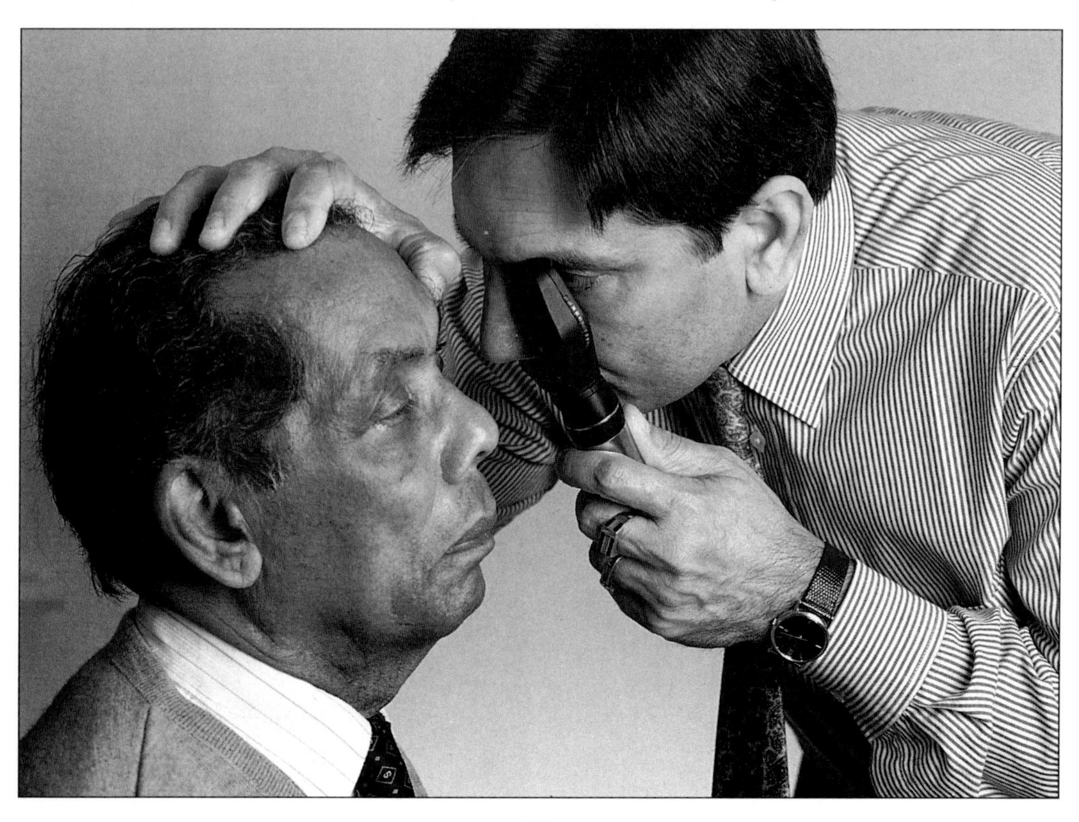

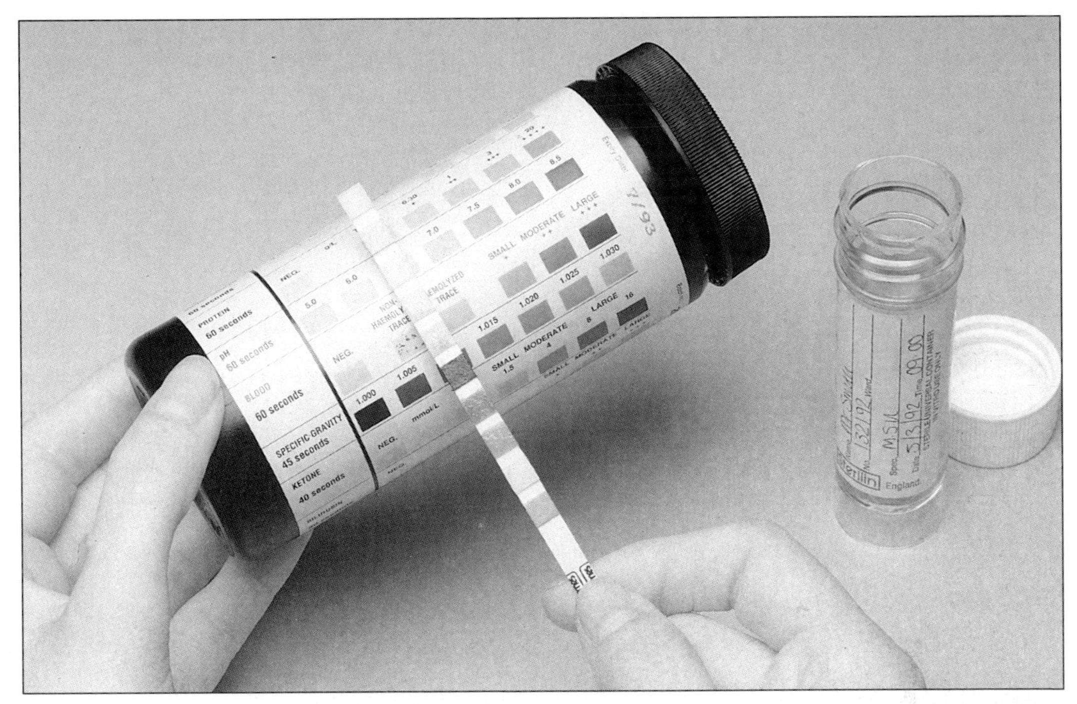

A urine test can be carried out to test for sugar in the urine. Usually a strip of special paper is placed in the urine and the subsequent colour change is noted.

results. If there is any doubt, you may be sent to a see a doctor at your local hospital to have the diagnosis confirmed. Children will usually go to someone with special expertise in looking after young people with this condition.

When the diagnosis is non-insulin dependent diabetes, it's more likely that most of your care will be in the hands of your doctor and his team, although you might need to go to the hospital diabetic clinic sometimes for particular problems or tests.

Some people with suspected diabetes may need an extra test which will be done at the hospital. This is necessary if the blood glucose level is borderline. The test, known as a glucose tolerance test (or GTT), will usually be done at your local hospital. You will be asked not to eat or drink anything other than plain water from the midnight before the morning when it is to be done. Urine and blood samples will be taken when you arrive at the clinic, then you'll be given a sweet drink containing a measured amount of glucose. The tests will then be repeated at intervals of one and two and possibly four hours to see whether your body is dealing with the glucose you've absorbed in the normal way. If the glucose levels in your blood are found to be abnormal, this will confirm the diagnosis of diabetes.

What is diabetes?

Causes of diabetes

Nobody really knows exactly why diabetes develops and what its causes are - only that people with diabetes do not make sufficient insulin in their bodies. We all need insulin for the conversion of sugar into energy. Insulin is a hormone which is produced in the pancreas. When the blood sugar levels rise, e.g. after a meal, insulin is released and helps to prevent blood sugar becoming too high. If there is insufficient insulin or it isn't functioning properly, diabetes will be the result.

Causes of Type I diabetes

This is known as young people's or juvenile diabetes. It usually develops suddenly and the symptoms are severe. It affects three to four adults in every one thousand aged between twenty and forty years. It also affects about two children in every thousand. Young people with this type of diabetes tend to have a genetic tendency towards it. The insulin-producing cells in the pancreas are damaged or completely destroyed. We do not know exactly why this happens, but there are some factors which may be involved, such as the body's abnormal reaction against the insulin producing cells, or a viral or other infection causing damage to the cells.

Causes of Type II diabetes

Again, the cause is not known. However, we do know that some people are more likely to develop non-insulin dependent diabetes than others. People who are overweight are in a higher risk group as are family members where this type of diabetes is passed down between the generations.

It tends to affect middle-aged and older people, and, in fact, used to be referred to as 'maturity onset' diabetes. People with Type II diabetes have some insulin in their body although it is insufficient for the maintenance of good health.

Diabetes facts

Many people are amazed when they learn that they have diabetes. Their first reaction is "Why me?" They wonder what has caused it and what they may have done wrong. There are lots of common misconceptions about diabetes so to put your mind at rest, take note of the following facts:

- You cannot 'catch' diabetes from somebody else.
- Other people can't catch diabetes from you.
- It is not caused by eating too much sugar or the wrong foods.
- It is not caused by shock, although this may help to trigger it off faster in a person who already has failing insulin production.
- Stress may exacerbate diabetes although it is not believed to cause it.
- Doctors do not think that diabetes can

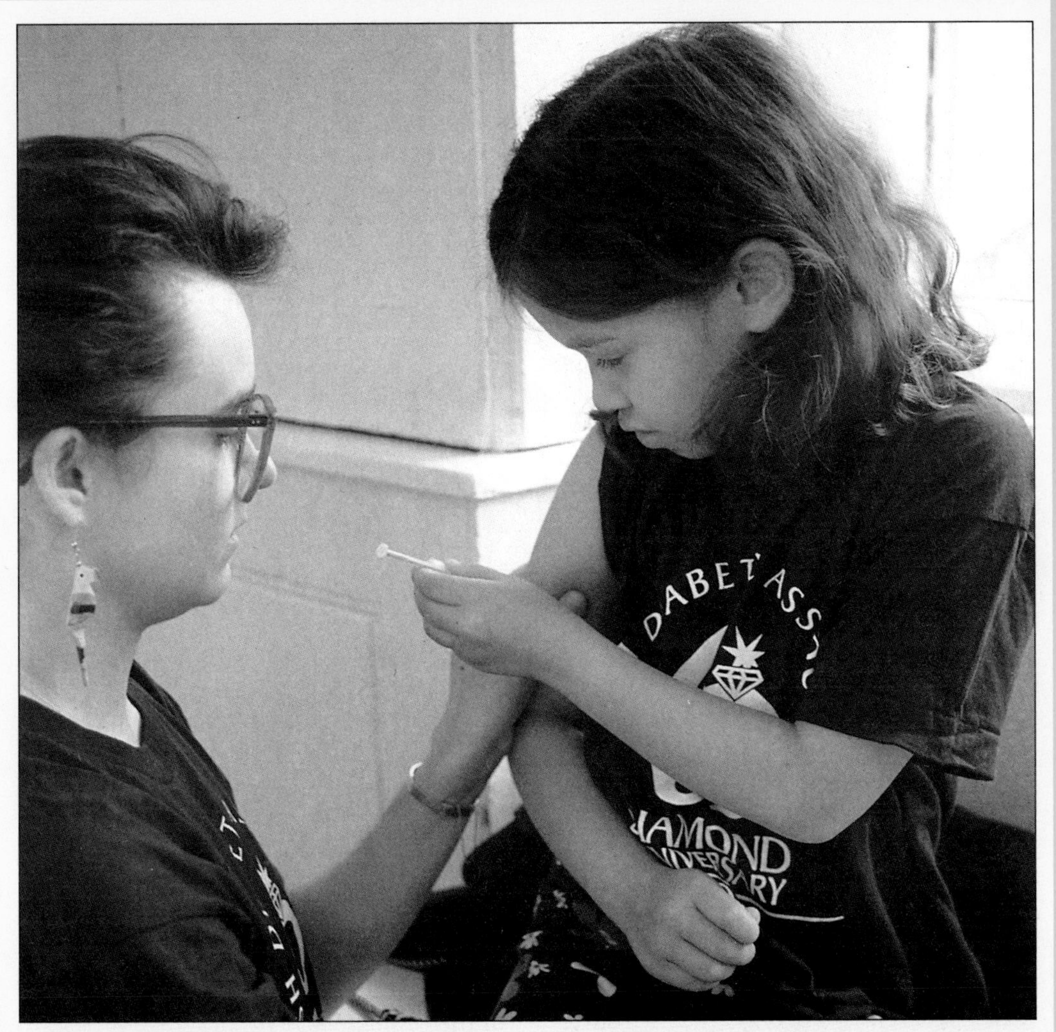

be caused by serious accidents or illnesses but they may lead to a temporary increase in blood sugar levels and thereby reveal that the person already had diabetes.

- Sometimes, although rarely, diabetes can be caused by diseases of the pancreas, e.g. pancreatitis in which the pancreas becomes inflamed.
- There is no 'cure' for diabetes, but you can learn to live with it and control it in such a way that you can lead a normal healthy life.

Chapter two

Treatment

Now that you know

Once you have been given a diagnosis, at least you know why you have been feeling unwell and can begin to get yourself on the road back to good health. Nevertheless, the implications are bound to take some time to sink in. It will be difficult to get all your questions together and new ones will crop up all the time. And of course it can be

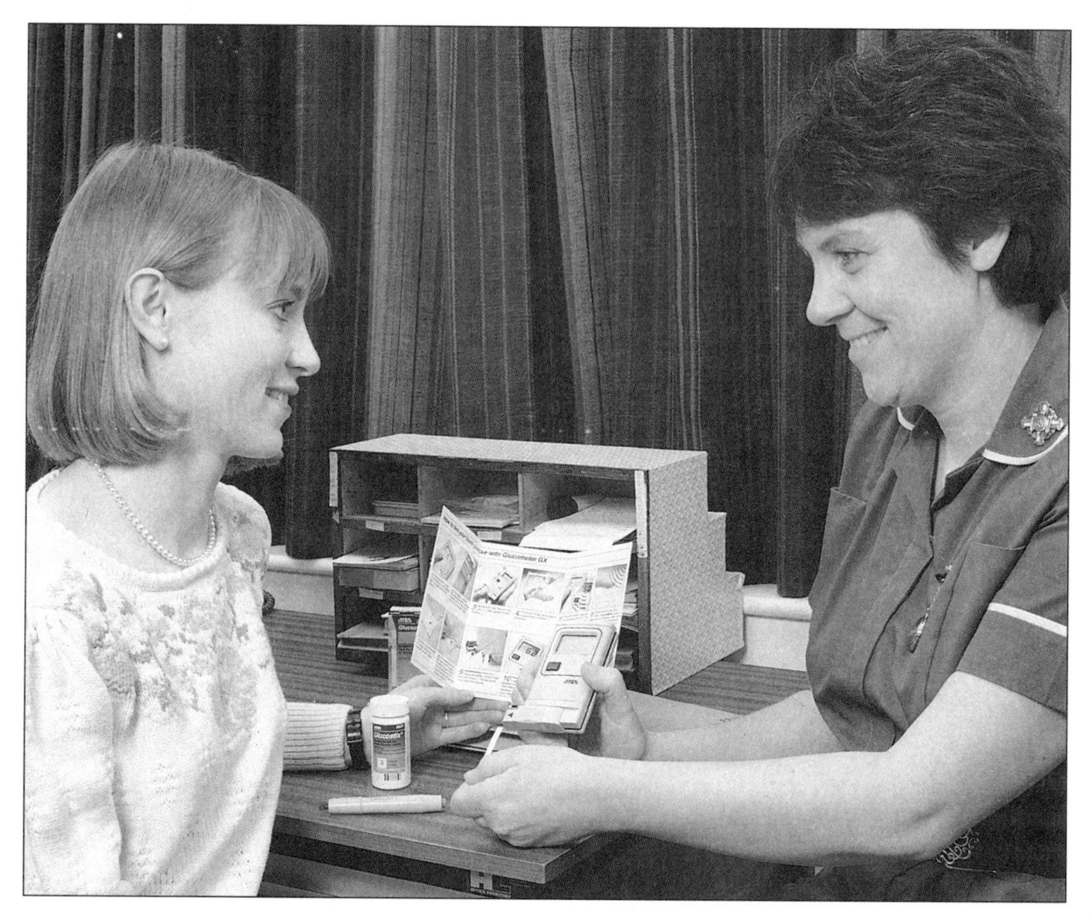

even harder to absorb all the information you'll be given regarding your diabetes and its treatment.

As insulin-diabetes can develop very quickly, some people will have symptoms which have become serious and need sorting out in hospital, so they may be admitted for a while. In some areas, this 'stabilization', as it's called, can be done in the patient's own home by a diabetes specialist nurse, in conjunction with the consultant and the diabetes team in the hospital.

People with Type II diabetes will probably not see a hospital consultant at this stage although they may do so later if they are one of the minority who need treatment with insulin. Your doctor will then be the person who'll explain the treatment and answer your questions, and you may see the practice nurse and dietitian as well.

More and more doctors now run regular diabetes clinics, but if yours doesn't or you feel your questions and worries haven't been dealt with satisfactorily, you can ask your doctor to refer you to a hospital diabetic clinic for more detailed advice.

Starting treatment

Regardless of which type of diabetes you have, part of your treatment will involve concentrating on healthy eating, which might mean a lot of changes for some people, depending on what your diet was like before. This sounds an alarming prospect, and one of your major concerns may well be that your days of enjoying your food are gone for good. In fact, this is far from the truth and there's absolutely no reason why you shouldn't have delicious meals and still eat in a healthy way.

In general, the sort of diet which experts now recommend follows the same principles of healthy eating which everyone would benefit from adopting. It means eating plenty of carbohydrates and fibre-rich foods, but keeping fat and sugar to a minimum. This may sound depressing, but it actually means you can have fresh vegetables, fruit and salad, brown bread and lots of high-fibre breakfast cereals, pulses like lentils and peas, fish of all kinds, wholemeal pasta and loads more delicious things. Like the rest of the population, you should cut down on foods that are high in animal fat, such as butter

Healthy eating tips

- Substitute skimmed or semi-skimmed milk for whole milk.
- Eat more unrefined carbohydrates and high-fibre foods, e.g. wholemeal bread, whole-grain breakfast cereals, brown rice, wholemeal pasta, fruit and vegetables.
- Use low-fat spread instead of butter.
- Eat more poultry and fish, and less red meat.
- Eat less sugar, e.g. cakes, sweets, chocolate, biscuits, sweetened drinks.

Treatment

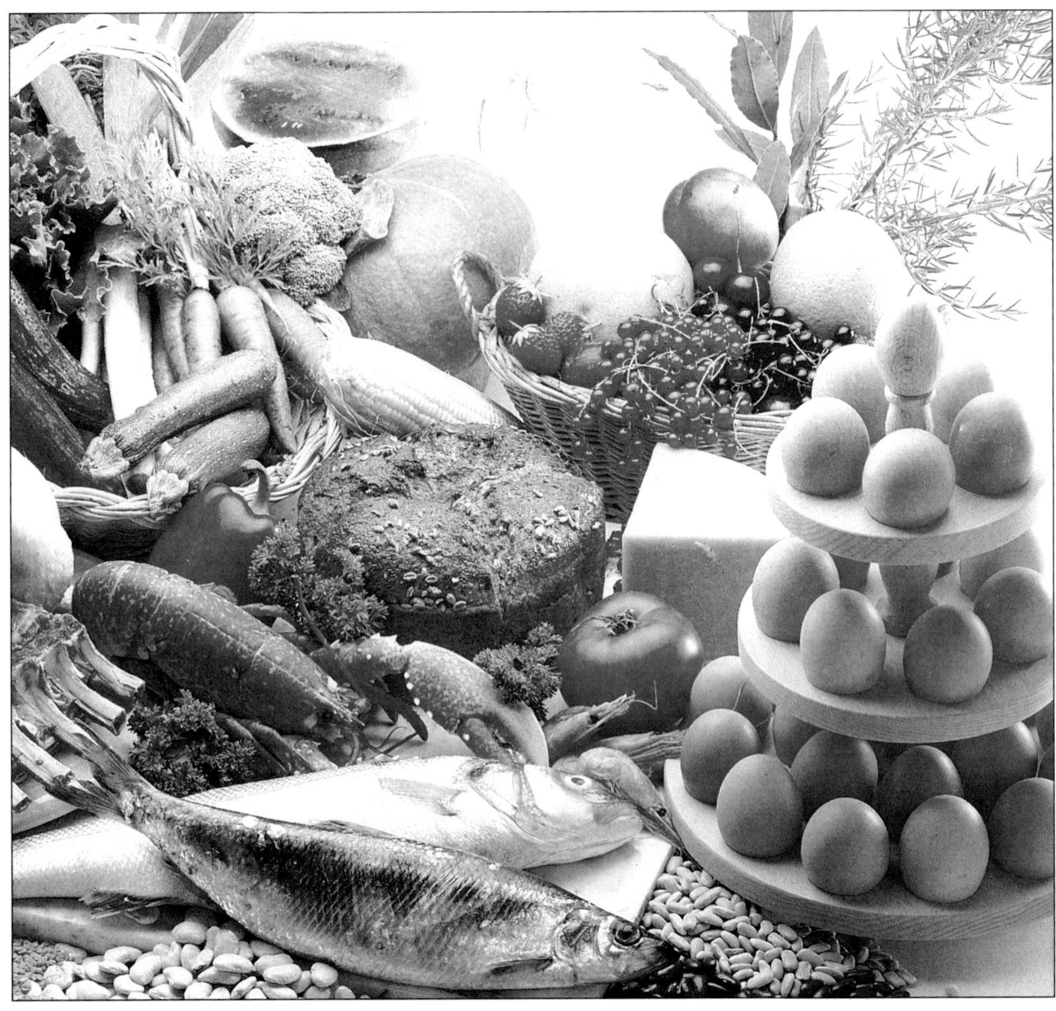

and cream, and keep fatty meats pretty low down on the menu. Not only will this new kind of diet be good as far as your diabetes is concerned, but it will also have lots of other health benefits. Many fruit and vegetables, for example, contain vitamins called anti-oxidants which may help protect you against heart disease and some forms of cancer, while fish – especially oily ones like salmon, trout, herrings and mackerel – contain substances which help maintain healthy joints and a healthy heart.

You don't need to eat a special diet, you just need to adopt a more healthy way of eating, especially fresh fruit, vegetables, whole-grain bread and cereals, beans and pulses.

People who follow these recommendations are very rarely overweight, so you shouldn't have to think about going on a slimming diet again once you've adapted your eating habits, although eating too much of any food can make you put on weight! When non-insulin dependent diabetes is newly diagnosed, you should be asked to concentrate on eating in a healthy way for six weeks. Later, you may need to go on tablets as well (see below). In any case, everyone with diabetes of whichever type will need to eat healthily for the rest of their lives. You will be given detailed advice by a dietician if necessary, and there are several excellent books and leaflets published to give the cook inspiration.

When you have to take tablets

There are different types of tablets which may be prescribed to help control your blood sugar levels and which are known as Oral Hypoglycaemic Agents (or OHAs):

- **Sulphonylureas (SUs)** – there are various different ones, but they all work by stimulating the pancreas to produce insulin.
- **Biguanides** – a drug called metformin stops the body from producing more sugar from other food and makes the insulin do its job more effectively.
- **Acarbose** – a relatively new drug which slows down the rate at which sugar enters the bloodstream.

Any of these tablets may be taken alone or in combination, depending on what suits the individual best. A few people do have side effects with these drugs, but your doctor should warn you what to watch out for. The main problem you might encounter when taking the SUs (but not when taking metformin or acarbose alone) is a hypoglycaemic episode or 'hypo', which is when your blood sugar level drops too far. The reason is usually that you have not eaten soon enough after taking your tablet, or that your dosage needs reducing, or that you have used up an unusual amount of energy. For more about this, see the section on page 53. People who are taking metformin tablets may suffer from stomach upsets such as diarrhoea and nausea. You will probably find this less of a problem if you take your tablets either with or immediately after meals, but if not, you should discuss it with your doctor.

Many people will find that taking tablets and following a suitable diet will together give them satisfactory control of their condition, but this system doesn't always work for everyone. If your home urine or blood tests show that your glucose readings are getting higher, despite taking the tablets and eating healthily, you should go back to your doctor. You may be one of the minority of people with NIDDMM who need insulin injections to control your diabetes.

When you need insulin injections

A minority of people with Type II and everyone with Type 1 diabetes will have to give themselves insulin by injection every day to control their blood glucose levels. The prospect is alarming and upsetting to many people, but the reality is much less daunting once you get over the initial shock.

The aim of the treatment is to mimic as closely as possible the insulin release pattern of someone who doesn't have diabetes. This is not as easy as it might sound, because the body is very clever at making subtle adjustments to insulin levels depending on the amount of glucose entering the bloodstream and the amount of energy being used. It is not easy to achieve this kind of variation when giving insulin artificially.

In an effort to tackle this problem, different kinds of insulin which take effect at different rates have been developed. All may be prepared from animals – pork and beef – or genetically engineered from human sources and have to be injected because insulin is a protein which would be destroyed by the digestive system if swallowed. Most people will need to have twice daily injections, but your doctor and specialist nurse will work out with you which 'regimen', i.e. which type, timing and dosage – meets your individual requirements best. It may be necessary to make some adjustments from time to time, perhaps to the type or the combination of insulin or even to the number of daily injections – to fit in with your lifestyle. You will have the opportunity

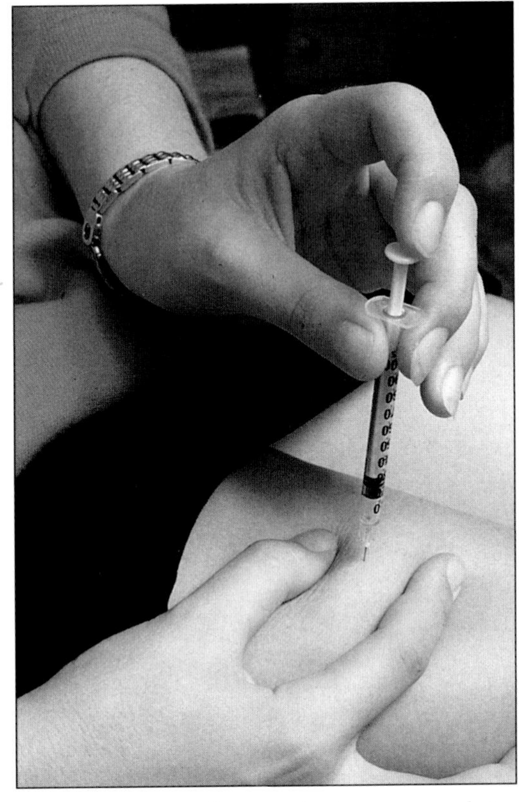

to discuss this with your doctor or specialist nurse at regular intervals, and you should certainly talk to them if you are concerned.

You probably find the idea of giving yourself injections quite worrying – if not positively frightening! Don't despair – you will be given as much help and instruction as you need and before long you will be doing the necessary without a second thought. The needles are very fine and you don't, as some people imagine, have to find a vein to insert

continued on page 24

Injection sites

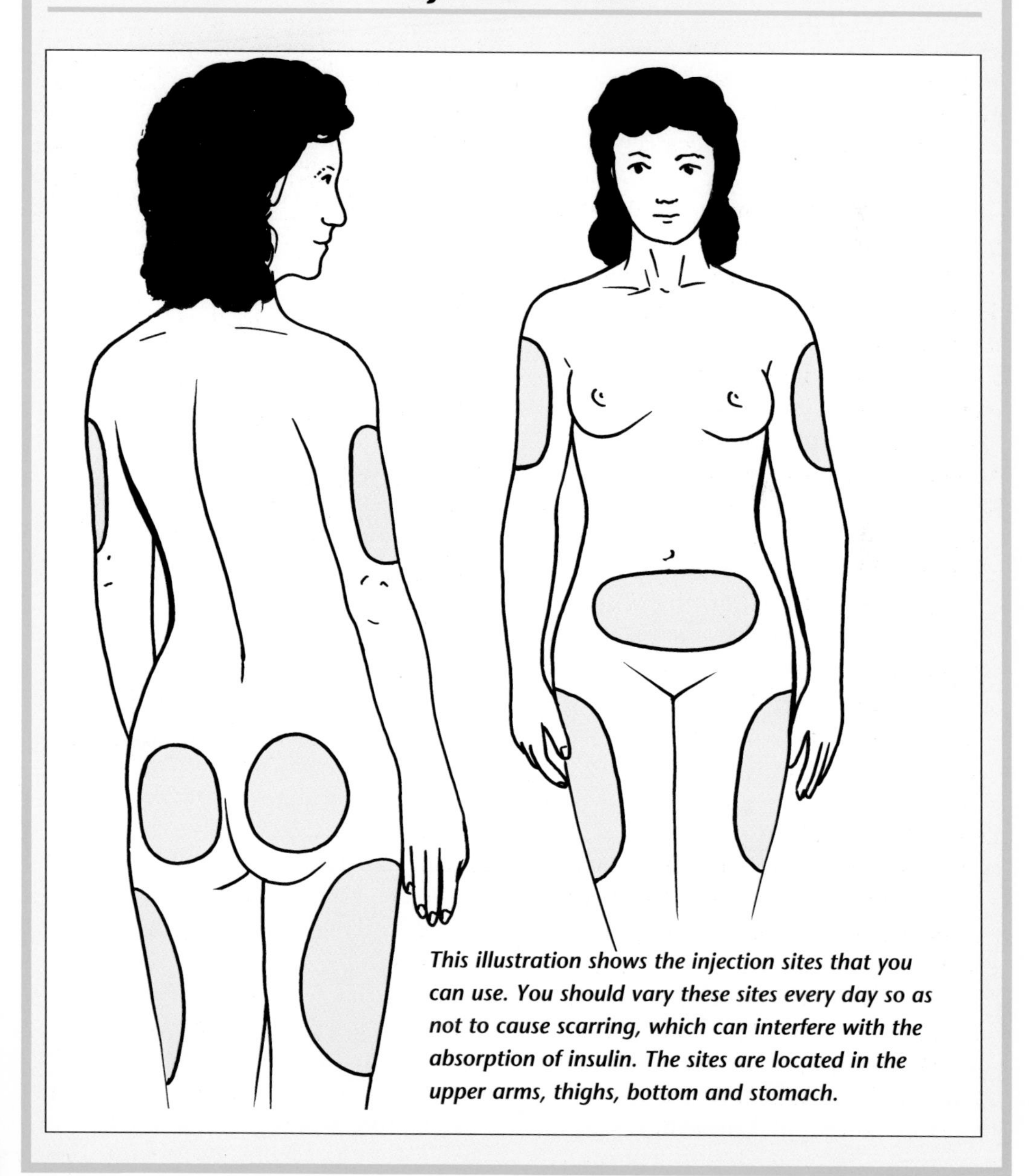

This illustration shows the injection sites that you can use. You should vary these sites every day so as not to cause scarring, which can interfere with the absorption of insulin. The sites are located in the upper arms, thighs, bottom and stomach.

Injecting insulin

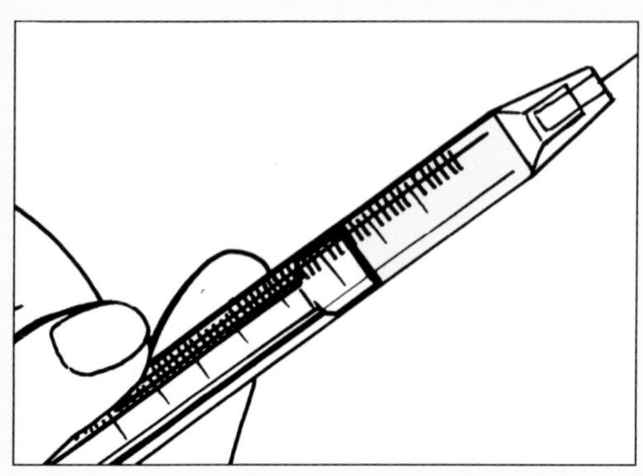

1 The way you draw up insulin into the syringe will vary according to the type of syringe and the type of insulin you use. Ask your doctor or specialist nurse to show you the correct procedure. It is very important that you are shown how to inject insulin before doing it yourself. Before you inject the insulin, be sure to check that you have drawn up the correct dose of insulin into the syringe.

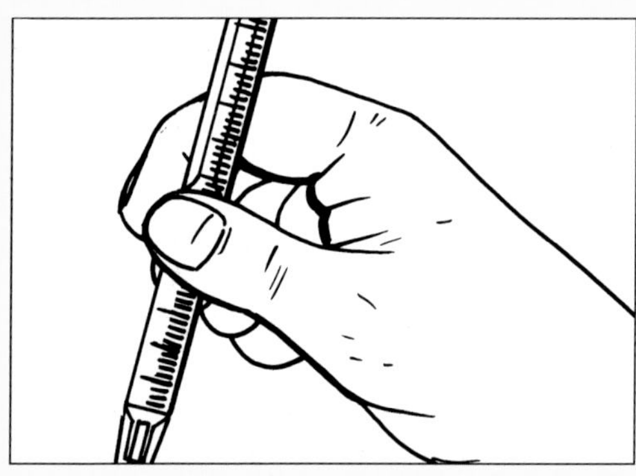

2 Hold the syringe pointing downwards (as shown here) but do not touch the tip of the needle which must be kept sterile.

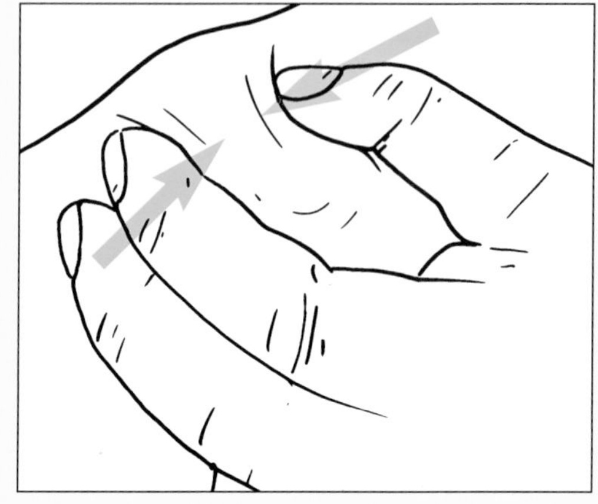

3 Prepare the injection site for the insulin injection. If there is not much flesh you will have to take the skin between your forefinger and thumb and pinch up a small mound.

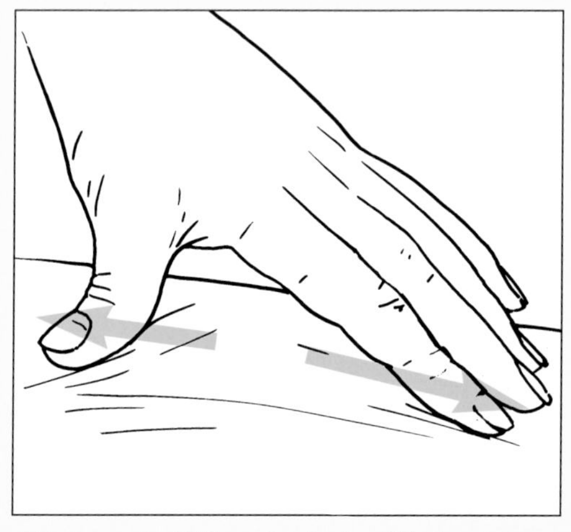

4 Conversely, if there is plenty of flesh, you must stretch out the skin between your forefinger and thumb.

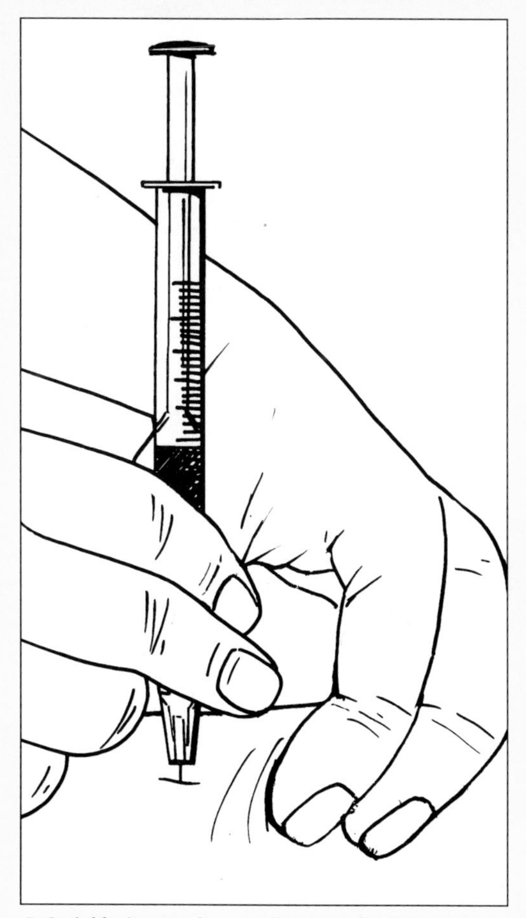

5 Quickly insert the needle straight into the skin. With practice, you will soon learn to do this painlessly and to the right depth. It is important that it penetrates below the skin, although it must not go too deep. Ask your doctor or nurse to show you.

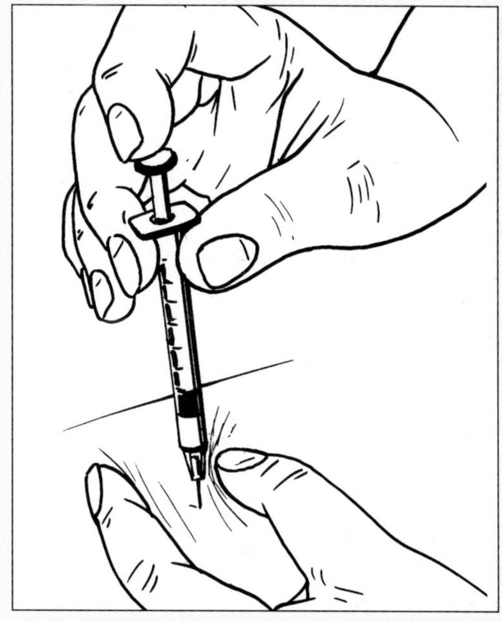

6 Hold the syringe steady while you press in the plunger with the other hand. Try to avoid any jerky movements and to keep the action smooth and fast.

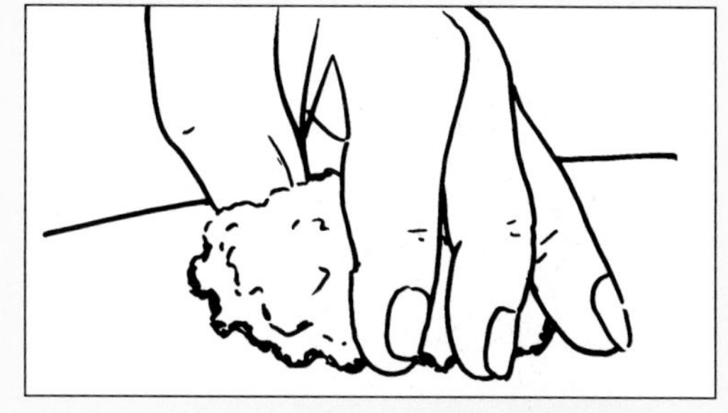

7 Quickly and smoothly pull out the needle, and then put some clean cotton wool or a tissue over the skin and press it down firmly. There is no need to hold it there for long: just a few seconds.

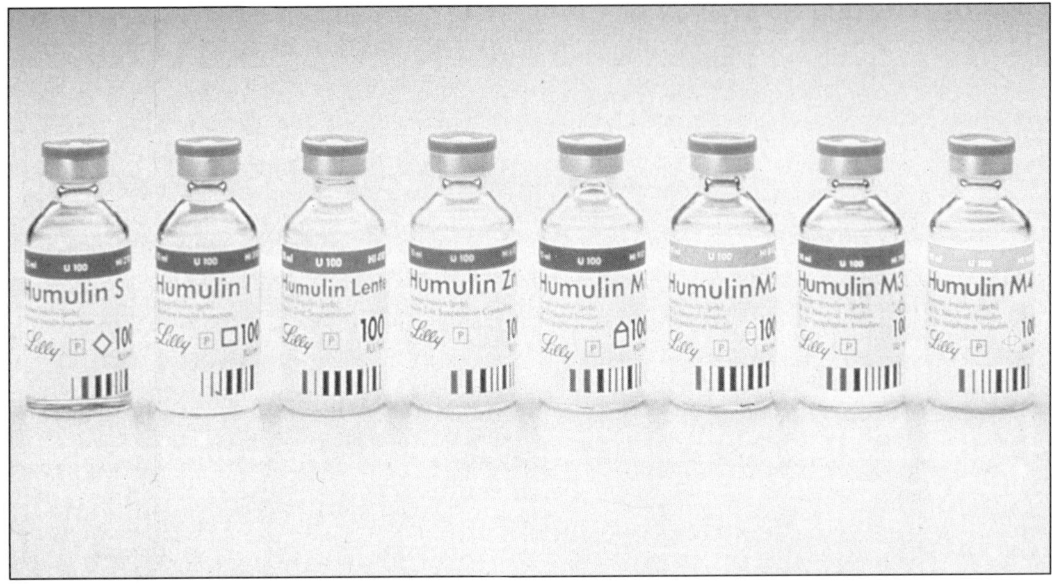

them into. The injection is done into an area where there is plenty of fat under the skin, such as the upper arms, thighs, stomach, bottom and calves. If you find injecting is painful at first, try numbing the area for 15 to 20 seconds by rubbing ice on the skin. This, and practice, should help, but if it doesn't, check with the specialist nurse who will be able to help you change your technique or find a better site for the injections.

Starting your new healthy eating plan

Unfortunately, neither tablets nor insulin injections alone are sufficient to keep diabetes under control. Their effect has to be backed up with a diet designed to keep your blood sugar level steady. If it is necessary for you to keep to a carbohydrate allowance, your doctor or dietician will explain how to do this, but otherwise it is a case of following a few relatively simple guidelines. Some people imagine that this will mean having different meals from the rest of the family or making a separate shopping list for 'diabetic' foods, but this is not true. Many people who develop NIDDMM are advised to lose weight when they are first diagnosed, and if this applies to you, you will be given advice on a healthy slimming diet.

Anyone who's always eaten a lot of fried foods, for example, or who has a sweet tooth may have a bit of a struggle learning to make do with less of them, but the good news is that your overall health, and that of your family, will be much better for the change.

The British Diabetic Association (BDA)

has devised some simple recommendations as described in the box on this page.

These days, you don't have to go to special 'health food' shops to find the kind of foods which will be part of your new way of eating: supermarket shelves are crammed with high-fibre foods such as wholewheat pasta, bread and flour, wholegrain and fibre–enriched cereals, low-fat yoghurts and alternatives to butter. Even with ready-made foods, you can easily find low-sugar, low-salt versions which taste just as good as the 'real thing'.

Sugary foods cause a rapid rise in blood sugar, so you really do have to cut down, but you don't have to renounce them for ever if you don't want to. Just remember to keep them as special treats, and have them after a meal rather than on an empty stomach. There's no reason why you shouldn't have artificial sweeteners in tea or coffee, but you can continue to use small amounts of ordinary sugar for making cakes and biscuits provided you don't do it too often! Experts agree that specially made 'diabetic' chocolates and other products are a waste of money and, anyway, they are usually no lower in fat or calories than the 'ordinary' equivalents.

Healthy eating guidelines

- It is important that you eat regular meals which are timed in relation to your insulin injections. Don't skip meals.
- Avoid being overweight. By eating a healthier diet which is low in fat, you should stabilize your weight.
- Eat more high-fibre carbohydrate foods, e.g. whole-grain cereals and bread.
- Eat less sugar and sugary foods.
- Cut down on the amount of fat you consume, and watch out for hidden fats in snack and convenience foods like biscuits, crisps, mayonnaise etc.
- Watch your salt intake - reduce the amount you use in cooking.
- Drink alcohol in moderation (see page 28 for guidelines).
- Avoid special diabetic products.

Slowly does it

For those people who face the prospect of a dramatic change to their eating pattern, the best approach is a gradual one. Start with the sort of changes which are easiest – swap to semi–skimmed milk, for example, and low-fat cheese and yoghurt instead of cream. Opt for wholemeal or granary bread, or at least the high-fibre white kind, and use low–fat spread instead of butter. Get into the habit of reading labels on food packaging – there are plenty of low-sugar jams, drinks, canned fruits and cereals around, and eating more fish and poultry (with the skin removed) will automatically reduce your fat intake.

In the UK the BDA has an excellent selection of leaflets and cookery books which will make adapting your diet a pleasure rather than a pain, and if you're at all confused about what to do, your dietitian will be happy to offer advice and practical tips to help you. Don't be afraid to ask questions of your dietitian or doctor.

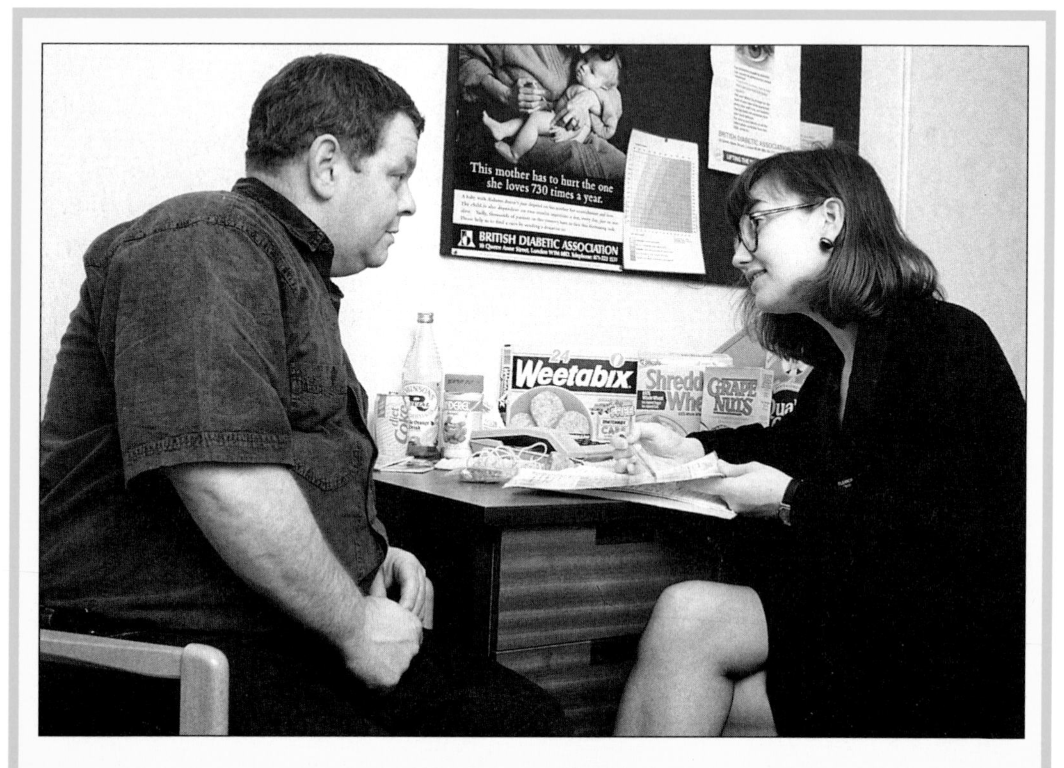

Consult a dietitian

You will probably be referred to a dietitian who will help you to plan out a healthy diet and advise on your daily calorie and carbohydrate intakes. You will be given specific advice which will take into account your own food preferences, circumstances, lifestyle and needs. You may also receive a diet sheet. If you are overweight, the dietitian may recommend that you should lose some weight. However, this must be done very carefully as dieting can affect the delicate balance between the insulin you inject and the blood sugar levels. Therefore your dietitian and doctor will have to plan a special weight-reducing diet for you.

Healthy eating

Your diet should reflect normal healthy eating principles, which are beneficial to everyone. Here are some basic guidelines for you to follow:

- Eat regular meals.
- Increase your consumption of high-fibre carbohydrate foods.
- Cut down on sugar.
- Eat less fat.
- Don't eat too much salt.
- Avoid special diabetic products.
- Keep alcohol to a minimum.

If you follow these recommendations you should stay relatively slim and healthy and avoid becoming overweight.

Calorie intake

You will be advised to keep your daily calorie intake reasonably constant and not to vary it too much. This will stabilize your weight and help you to control your diabetes. Your doctor or dietitian will advise on how many calories are best for you. Most fresh fruit and vegetables, whole-grain cereals, low-fat dairy products, white fish and poultry tend to be low to medium in calories and are very healthy options. Watch out for hidden calories in fried foods, fatty meat, cream, butter and full-fat cheeses, chocolate, pastry, sweets and sugary foods and drinks.

You should get at least fifty per cent of your calories every day from starchy carbohydrate foods. These include:

- Wholemeal bread.
- Whole-grain cereals, e.g. breakfast cereals.
- Potatoes.
- Beans, lentils and pulses.
- Wholemeal flour and pasta.
- Brown rice.

There are some foods that promote a slow, steady rise in blood glucose levels, and you should eat these regularly: oats, beans, lentils and citrus fruits, e.g. oranges and lemons.

More refined and sugary carbohydrate foods tend to be rapidly absorbed into the bloodstream, and these should be saved for special occasions, as a snack before strenuous exercise, or for emergencies, e.g. hypoglycaemia or illness. These foods include chocolate, sweets and sugary drinks.

Cut down on sugar

There are many ways in which you can reduce the sugar in your diet. Here are some tips to help you:

- Eat fruit which is canned in natural juice rather than syrup.
- Use an artificial sweetener rather than sugar for sweetening drinks and cereals.
- Choose reduced-sugar or pure fruit jams and spreads.
- Reduce the sugar you use in desserts and puddings; use artificial sweetener, or fresh or dried fruit instead.

Healthy eating

Cut down on fat

Reducing the fat in your diet will not only help you to control your calorie intake better and eat more healthily, but it will also help reduce the risk of heart disease.

- Eat more white fish and poultry and less fatty red meat.
- Substitute low-fat spreads for butter and margarine.
- Use skimmed or semi-skimmed milk, low-fat yogurt and cheeses.
- Remove the skin from poultry.
- Top desserts with yogurt instead of cream.
- Grill fish, meat and poultry instead of frying them.
- Use the minimum of oil or fat when making soups, stews and casseroles.
- Cut down on pastry, cakes, biscuits, potato crisps etc. which are all high in fat.

Eat less salt

It is sensible to eat less salt as a high intake may be a factor in high blood pressure. You can reduce the amount of salt in your diet by a few simple measures.

- Add less salt to food at the table.
- When cooking, use more natural seasonings, e.g. herbs and spices, and less salt.
- Eat fewer highly salted foods, e.g. smoked fish, preserved and pre-cooked meat products, hard cheeses, salted potato crisps, peanuts and many other snack and convenience foods.
- Read the labels carefully on canned products - many soups and canned vegetables are high in salt.

Alcohol in moderation

You should keep your alcohol consumption to a minimum and follow these standard guidelines after checking with your doctor first.

- Men can drink a maximum of three standard drinks a day.
- Women can drink a maximum of two standard drinks a day.

Note: One standard drink is equal to one of the following:

- 300ml/½ pint ordinary beer or lager.
- one single measure of spirits, e.g. gin, whisky, vodka, rum etc.
- One glass of dry white wine.
- One small glass of dry sherry.
- One measure of vermouth or a similar aperitif.

Remember that these are maximums, and it is better to drink less or avoid alcohol altogether. It is essential that you never drink on an empty stomach, as alcohol lowers blood sugar levels. Nor should you have a drink instead of a meal or snack.

Testing times

The measure of successful treatment of diabetes is the level of glucose in the blood, so learning to test this yourself is extremely valuable. Fortunately, scientists are constantly coming up with new and improved ways of doing this, and you don't need a degree in medicine or chemistry to master it.

There are two ways of testing the level of glucose in your blood – urine checks and blood tests. Many people with diabetes wonder why they can't simply rely on how they feel to assess whether their levels are too high or too low, and find frequent testing a chore. Unfortunately, the body is a bit slow about providing clues to blood glucose levels; they may often be well out of the acceptable range before you notice any ill effects.

Which test?

- Urine testing – using chemical test strips.
- Blood tests – using lancets and a special machine for pricking your finger, plus testing strips. You can also buy blood glucose meters over the counter in the drugstore for a more accurate result. Contact your diabetes nurse, specialist or doctor for information about them.

Urine checks

Some people with NIDDMM may be advised by their doctor to monitor their blood glucose levels by means of urine checks. You'll be prescribed special chemical test strips, and to start with you'll need to do the check every day. People are often told to do it just before breakfast, and this test should give a negative result. It is also useful to do it one to two hours after a main meal to assess your response to food. Eventually you will, it is hoped, find that you're getting negative results all the time, and if the clinic blood test confirms that your diabetes is under control, they may recommend that you only

Urine testing

There are many testing kits available for testing the amount of sugar in your urine. They are simple to use and usually involve either:

1 Observing the colour change when a tablet is added to the urine in a test tube, or

2 Observing the colour change when a strip of specially treated paper is quickly dipped in a stream of urine.

For accurate interpretation of the results of the test, you must know when you last passed urine as this will affect the sugar levels.

do the urine test about once a week.

The problem with urine testing is that your blood glucose level can be quite high before it shows up in your urine, and low levels won't be indicated at all. To complicate matters further, urine test readings can mean different things with different people. Some find that glucose leaks into their urine when their blood level is only slightly raised, while others can go on having negative urine tests even though their blood levels are raised quite a lot above normal. Doctors refer to this latter group as having a high renal threshold. The urine test only reflects what your blood glucose level was some hours before you did it.

Blood testing

SBGM (or self blood glucose monitoring as it is officially known) gives a much more accurate result than urine testing, and is the method used by the majority of people with diabetes.Your doctor or specialist nurse will show you how to do the test, and let you practise until you are confident. They will also tell you when is the best time to do it, and how often it needs to be repeated each day. This is likely to be less frequently for people with NIDDMM than for those taking insulin.

Each reading is a kind of snapshot showing the situation at the time you did the test. What you really need is more like a film record of your blood sugar levels throughout the day, and possibly the night too, especially if you have IDDM and are at risk of low blood sugar during the night. To build up this record, it is useful to carry out a series of tests during the day and occasionally at night, if necessary, so that you can build up a complete picture of what is happening to your blood sugar levels, and how it relates to your life – when you eat, take exercise, or your insulin dose, if relevant.

The right result

In an ideal world, your blood sugar readings would be between 3.5 and 8 mmol/l. In practice, this degree of accurate control may be difficult, especially at first, and provided your readings are generally below 10mmol/l you will be doing well. You will almost certainly have the odd 'rogue' reading when the level is unusually high. You should record it, but you don't need to take any action unless it happens on several consecutive tests.

What's the point?

Many people with diabetes dislike doing regular tests and are driven at times to wonder whether it's all really necessary. Others feel that it draws them into concentrating too much on their condition when what they want is to forget about it as much as possible and get on with their lives.

The way to counter these concerns is to recognise that the point of testing is to give you control over your diabetes and help you to stay in the best possible health. You're not testing and recording for the sake of it, but to provide the vital information about the way your body is responding which you and your doctor need to enable you to adjust your treatment to fit into your lifestyle so you can live normally without unnecessary worry.

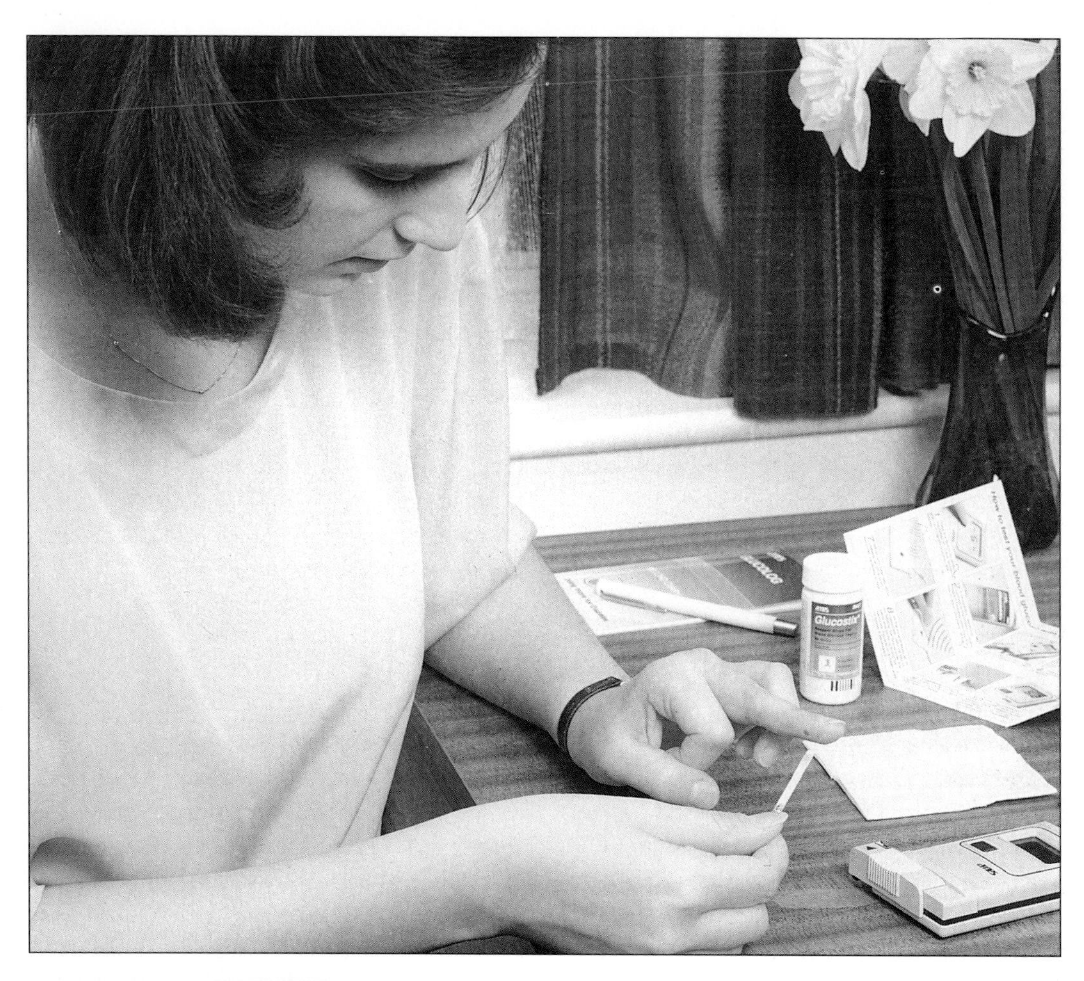

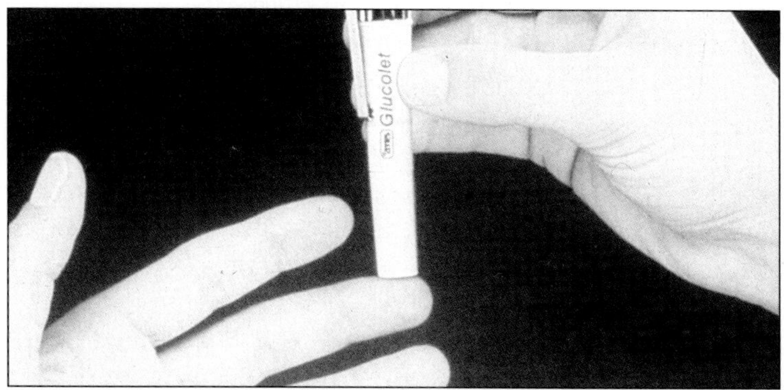

When obtaining a blood sample with a finger-pricking device, you should insert it on the side of the finger, not the tip. Our fingertips are very sensitive and easily become sore.

Treatment

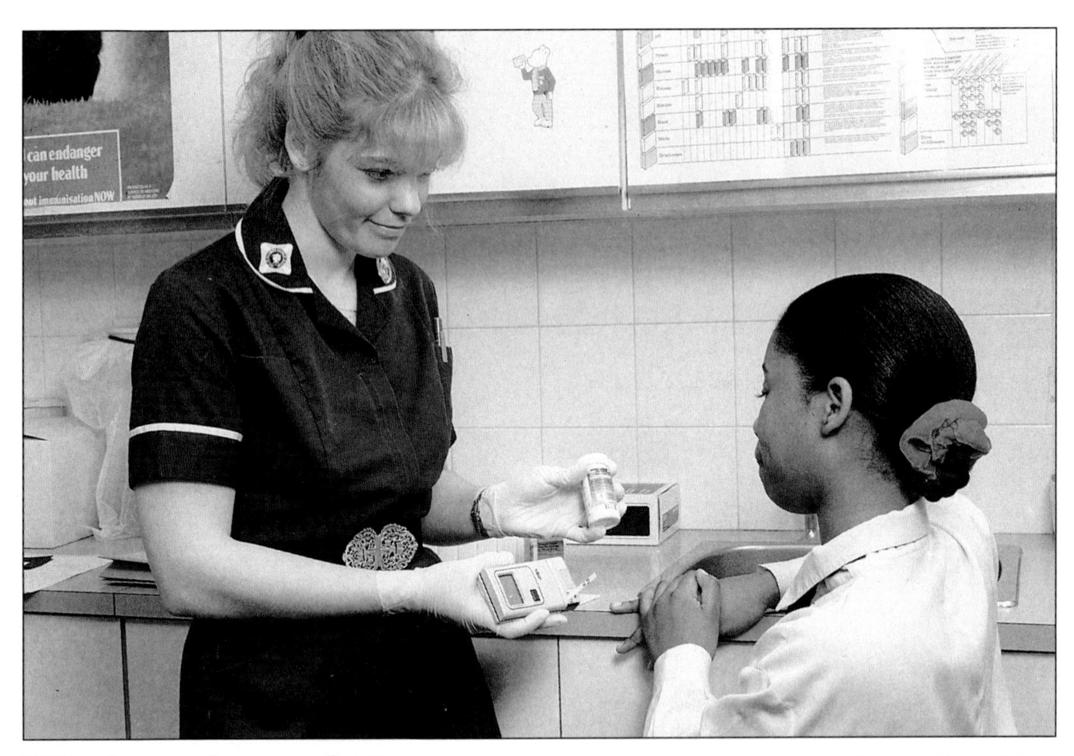

The specialist nurse or your doctor will explain to you how to obtain blood samples and also how to test them and monitor your blood glucose levels.

Practice makes perfect

The prospect of pricking your finger to draw blood several times a day is unappealing, but there are a variety of gadgets available designed to make the process as simple and painless as possible. You may need to talk to your doctor or specialist nurse who can advise you about how to do it successfully, and they will also show you the correct technique for taking a reading. The tips of your fingers are sensitive and may become sore, so to avoid this you may be advised to use the sides or wherever is most comfortable for you. You'll need practice too to make sure you're using the visual testing strips or blood glucose monitor correctly – poor technique will give misleading readings! Don't despair though – however hard it seems at first you will get the hang of it, and as you gain better control of your diabetes, you will reap the rewards in terms of a much greater sense of well-being.

Chapter three
Help is at hand

You will inevitably get to know the people involved in your care rather well over the weeks and months to come, and with luck a degree of mutual trust will be built up so that you will find it easy to raise any questions or worries which are on your mind. Depending on the individual, this may be mostly handled through a hospital clinic or your doctor's surgery. People who have just been diagnosed with IDDM may find that, initially at least, their treatment and care are arranged through the hospital clinic, although you may have the option of switching to a doctor's clinic later on. In any case, you may sometimes need to see other specialists concerned with particular aspects of your condition such as diet, eye care and detecting or treating any other complications, for example.

Doctors' clinics

Many practices in the UK run regular clinics for people with diabetes, sometimes in conjunction with a local hospital specialist who attends the clinic regularly to see patients. Where this does not happen, the practice will usually have a good relationship with the diabetes clinic staff at the hospital, to whom you may be referred if and when the need arises. Some doctors offer a system of 'shared care', which means that you will see a doctor at the hospital once a year while seeing your own doctor most of the time. Your doctor will almost certainly have a practice nurse working

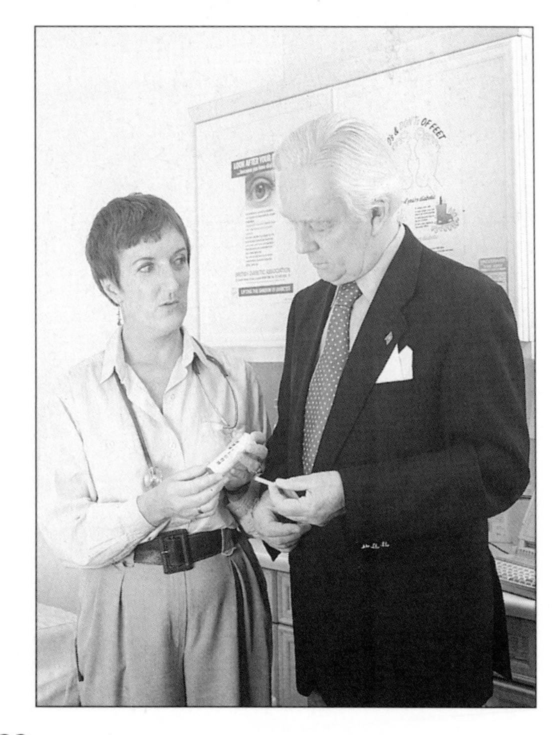

Your own doctor will probably handle most of your diabetes care, often with the help of a practice nurse or specialist nurse. Some doctors even run their own diabetes clinics, which may be attended by a consultant from the local hospital.

with him, and sometimes a chiropodist too, but you may have to go elsewhere to see other specialists such as a dietitian.

Not all family doctors take a special interest in diabetes and so may not offer a clinic service. In this case, you could consider changing to another doctor who does, but you may prefer to opt for a hospital clinic instead, while sticking with your regular doctor for all your other health needs.

Hospital clinics

You will meet (and be dealt with) by more people at a hospital clinic, and, of course, you may not always see the same doctor twice. However, you will find a wider range of services on offer, and there will also be other specialists at hand if you need them at any time. As well as the doctors, you will probably see the diabetes nurse specialist who will help you with any problems, teach you how to do blood or urine tests and give yourself insulin injections, if necessary, as well as providing all the information you need to enable you to live with your diabetes. She may also visit you at home, which can be a big plus if you're under the weather.

Another expert whose advice will be invaluable is the dietitian, and you will probably see her at regular intervals to make sure all is well or raise any problems. When

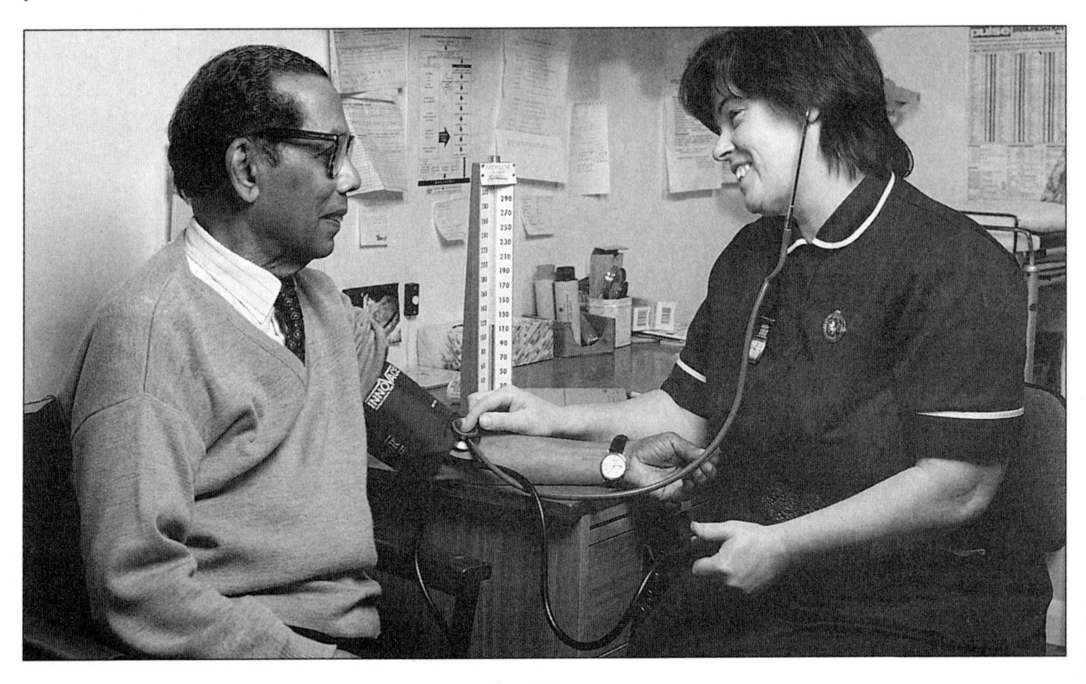

you are first diagnosed, you will probably also have an appointment with a chiropodist, as good foot care is very important for someone with diabetes. (For more on this, see page 58). Teamwork in diabetes care is essential, and all the specialists mentioned here will work within this team.

A family affair

When your diabetes is first diagnosed, your family will be at least as taken aback as you are, and will probably be worried not only about you, but also about the impact it will have on family life in general. Most doctors and specialist or practice nurses will be quite happy for you to ask a relative to come with you when you have an appointment. It is useful for them to understand what your treatment will involve, to know about testing and to discuss the implications of any changes to your diet. The dietitian in particular can be a great help in explaining that your diet doesn't mean separate meals or misery all round. Obviously, it is much easier to continue to eat healthily if those you share meals with do so too. And, of course, there's no doubt that they would be giving their own health a boost by eating the way you do.

If you have IDDM or are taking tablets which might mean you have hypoglycaemic episodes, you and your family should also know about any signs to watch for and what to do about it (see page 53). The more they understand, the less anxious they will be, and they will also be able to give you moral and practical support while you're learning to cope with your diabetes.

The same applies to some extent to other

The British Diabetic Association

However knowledgeable and sympathetic your medical advisers, you may sometimes feel that they can't possibly understand what it really feels like to have diabetes. Talking to other people who have gone through the same experience can be very encouraging and reassuring, and you may learn a lot by finding out how they've coped. In the UK, the BDA has 400 branches all round the country, which as well as being a great source of information and support can also be great fun.

Even if you don't feel ready to take part to that degree, it really is worthwhile becoming a member of the BDA. Their range of books, leaflets, information packs and videos covers just about everything you could possibly want to know. If you need the answer to a particular query which isn't covered, they have experts who will be able to help either by phone on the 'Care Line' or by letter.

Help is at hand

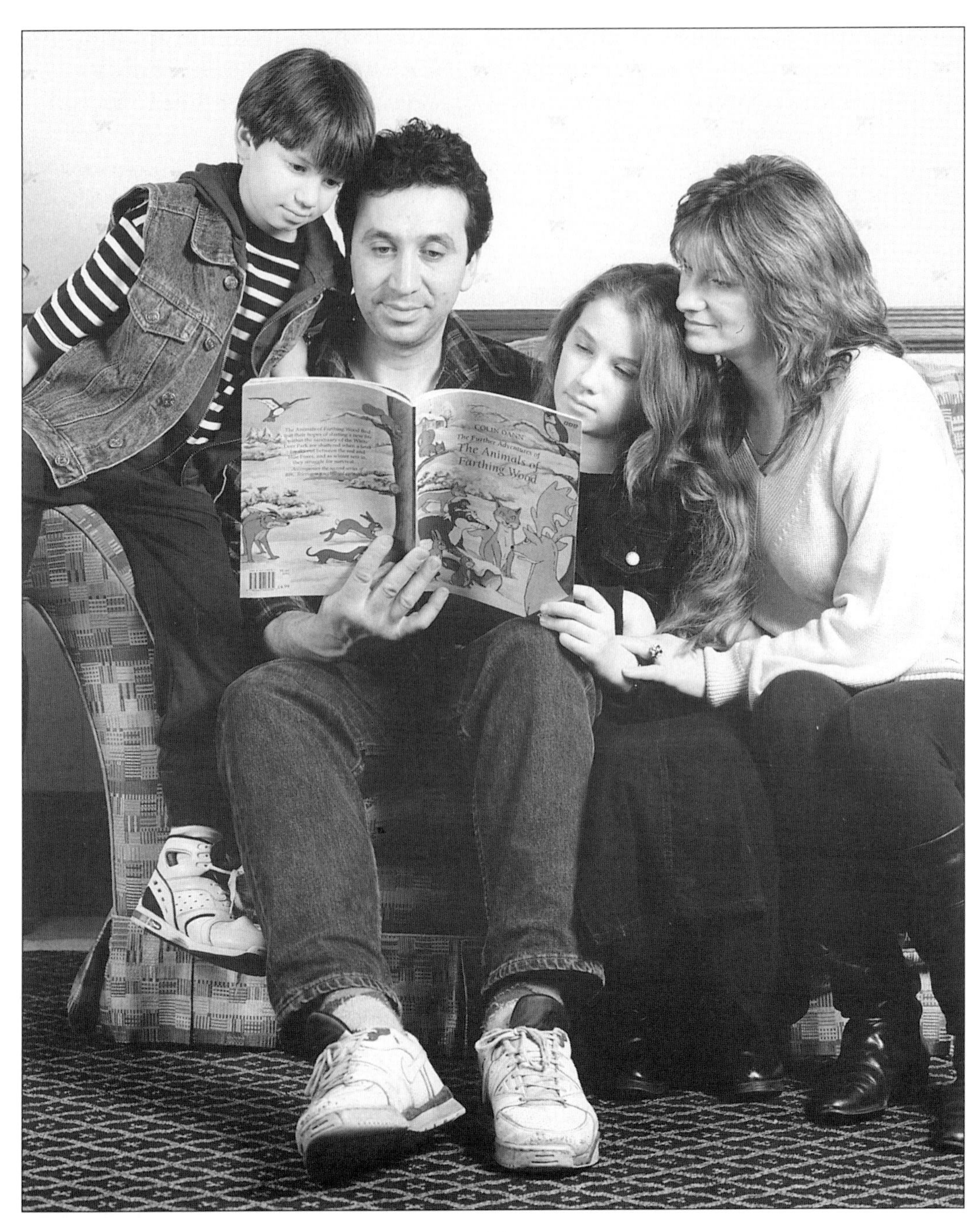

people you spend a lot of time with – your close work colleagues, classmates or fellow students and teachers. While you probably won't want to broadcast your health details to the world, other people will be more supportive if you tell them something about what having diabetes means. For example, they may need to know that a meeting which runs on through lunchtime could be a real problem – rather than just a minor irritation – for you, or that there are good reasons why it's not a good idea for you to join in an after hours drinking session with just a few crisps to keep you going. You might also feel you want to warn them about the possibility of hypoglycaemic episodes, again so they can be aware of signs and know what action needs to be taken.

As well as reading this book, you will probably be looking for other sources of information, and you may want to suggest that family and close friends have a read through some of the material available through the BDA.Their members' magazine, *Balance* makes especially interesting reading, even if you haven't got diabetes yourself, and often has features especially for families and friends of people with diabetes. The BDA also produces two free magazines designed for people with newly–diagnosed insulin– and non–insulin, dependent diabetes called *Balance for Beginners* which are packed with useful information and advice.

Everyone will find their own balance between telling other people what they need to know and sharing the details of their medical history with all and sundry. In any case, once you yourself have got used to coping with your diabetes, you'll find that most people take their cue from you. If you don't make a fuss about diabetes, they probably won't either.

Family life

It will help you to control your diabetes better and live a normal active life if your family understand what is involved and offer you practical and moral support. It is particularly important that other family members learn to recognise the warning signs of a hypo, and how to treat it when it occurs.

To avoid cooking separate meals, it is a good idea if they adopt your healthier way of eating. They will soon feel the benefits of this. They can also give encouragement and support by embarking on an exercise regime with you, perhaps by going for a walk or a cycle together at weekends, or going swimming or joining your local health club or fitness centre.

Children with diabetes

It is not only adults who develop diabetes; children may be affected, too. In fact, it is estimated in the UK that one in every 500 schoolchildren has diabetes. Many parents find it difficult to comprehend and accept that their child is diabetic. They are particularly alarmed when they realise that there is as yet no cure and it is a condition that the child will have to live with for the rest of his life. The idea of giving injections to their child is also a horrifying one.

It is important that your child should lead as normal a life as possible: going to school, playing with his friends and joining in with his peers in games, sport and activities. Ensure that he eats a healthy diet with adequate carbohydrate. Your doctor or dietitian can answer any queries you may have on this. Most school meals are nutritionally well balanced and are suitable for your child. However, if you are worried that he might not receive the right food or may make the wrong choices (if the school operates a cafeteria system), then you may have to talk to the teachers or provide a packed lunch each day.

Diabetes and school

You should inform the school and all your child's teachers that he has diabetes, and ensure that they know what to do in the event of a hypo. If necessary, write down any special information they might need, e.g. warning signs and treatment of a hypoglycaemic reaction, and any dietary information.

Teachers should appreciate the following points:

- It is often better to give a child some sugar lumps or a biscuit if he has a hypo rather than sending him home from school.
- The child should take extra carbohydrate before exercise or games. He should be encouraged to participate in sport as there is no reason why he should not compete even at the highest level.
- The child will need regular meals and should not be permitted to miss these or to eat at unusual times. He may also need a snack in the middle of the morning and afternoon.
- If your child needs to perform urine tests or blood tests at school, it should be possible to do so in privacy and comfort away from other children, which can be embarrassing.
- It should be possible to perform injections at home in the morning and evening, thereby avoiding the necessity of injecting at school. However, if your child goes away to camp or on a school trip, he may have to take his insulin with him. If so, make sure that your child is capable of injecting himself or that there is a teacher or adult who can do it for him. You will need to brief teachers about the correct insulin dosage and the times at which injections should be given.

Insulin injections

Ideally, children should learn as soon as possible how to inject themselves. Many children as young as six or seven years old can do this under parental supervision. They should certainly be able to do it by the time they are eleven years of age and starting senior school. It is always a good idea for an adult to check that the correct dosage of insulin is being administered and that it has been drawn up properly.

Hypoglycaemia in children

Talk to your doctor about recognising the warning signs and learn how to deal with a hypoglycaemic reaction should it occur. Some of the symptoms to look out for are as follows:

- Tearfulness for no apparent reason.
- Lack of energy and listlessness.
- Inability to concentrate.
- Sweating and unusually pale skin.
- In schoolchildren, reading difficulties and finding it hard to answer questions.
- Hunger.
- Feeling shaky.
- Headache or double vision.

This may lead to vomiting, convulsions and even unconsciousness, in which case you must always seek medical help immediately. Important: if the child is conscious, you should give him sugar immediately. Offer three sugar lumps or two heaped teaspoons of sugar in water, or some glucose tablets to suck. The child should recover quickly and he should then eat a biscuit or a starchy snack, such as a sandwich.

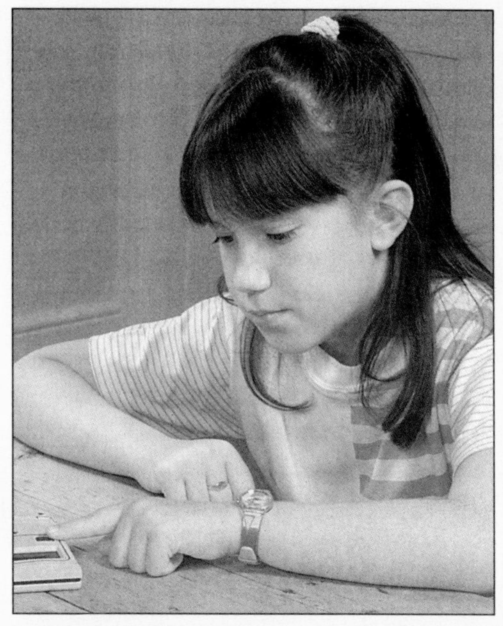

Important: if the child is unconscious or having a fit, it is impossible to administer sugar by mouth. However, the body will produce its own sugar and within a few minutes the child should recover and be able to take some sugar in a glass of water. If he does not recover, contact the doctor immediately. Try to keep calm and not to worry. Hypoglycaemia in children cannot cause brain damage or death as many parents fear, nor will it affect the child's physical and intellectual development.

Help is at hand

Help yourself

While you might prefer to ignore your diabetes as far as possible and certainly don't want it to dominate your life, it really is worth learning as much about it as you can. By keeping a careful note of your home blood glucose test results and relating this information to your own lifestyle, you will be able to find the best way of living with your diabetes. Through discussion with your medical advisers, you will be able to ensure that your treatment is tailored as precisely as possible to your needs. No two people with diabetes are exactly alike, so there's a lot you can do to help your diabetes team to help you. Their care of you is bound to be dependent to a considerable extent on the information you can give them, so never be afraid to speak up and give your point of view.

Most people, whether or not they have diabetes, would benefit from adopting a healthier lifestyle. When you do have this condition, however, you have an even greater incentive to get rid of bad habits and take positive steps to improve your overall health.

- Your new way of eating will make it easier

Home testing

You can monitor your blood glucose levels and keep your diabetes under control by regular testing. Your doctor will advise you on how often you should do this. Blood glucose meters are small, compact and easy to use, and give fast, accurate results.

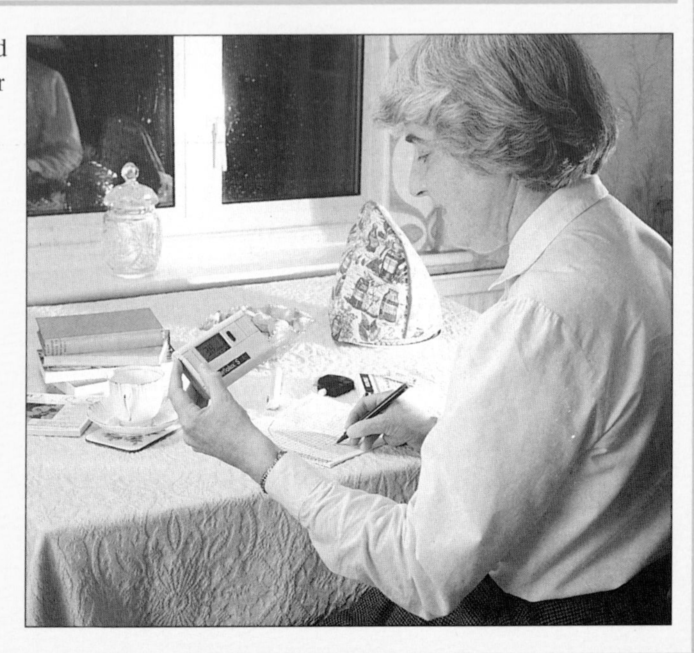

Alcohol

The good news for those who like a drink is that you don't have to give up alcohol. However, like the rest of the population, you should limit yourself to no more than two drinks a day if you're a woman, and three if you're a man. Experts talk in terms of 'units of alcohol' – one unit is the equivalent of half a pint of beer, a single measure of spirits or a small glass of wine or sherry, for example. Beware of the calories contained in alcohol, especially if you are overweight, and try to have a couple of days each week without any alcohol at all. Try not to drink on an empty stomach as it lowers your blood sugar level, and you should never be tempted to have a drink instead of a meal. Low-alcohol beers are fine, provided you remember that they contain quite a lot of sugar, but steer clear of the low-carbohydrate or low-sugar beers as they are high in alcohol.

If you take insulin or sulphonylurea tablets, make sure you don't drink on an empty stomach. Have an extra snack if it's not time for your next meal. People who have never seen the symptoms of a hypo (see page 53) may just think you're drunk, so make sure there's someone with you who would know what to do if necessary, and carry something with you which will let people know you have diabetes if they are trying to help you.

Guidelines for alcohol consumption

Men: They may drink a maximum of three standard drinks a day(see below).
Women: They may drink a maximum of two standard drinks a day(see below).

As a guide, one standard drink is equal to one of the following:

- A 300ml/½ pint glass of ordinary beer or lager.
- One single measure of spirits, e.g. gin, whisky, vodka, rum.
- One regular glass of dry white wine.
- One small glass of dry sherry.
- One measure of vermouth or a similar aperitif.

to stabilize your weight at a level which is right for your height and build. However, if you do need to shift a few pounds – or even stones – arrange to talk to the dietitian who can help you do this safely and without too much self-denial.

- Smoking is even more dangerous for someone with diabetes than for the rest of the population because it increases the chances of developing heart disease or kidney problems. Knowing just how much you have to gain by giving up is the first step on the road to success – but if you feel you can't manage to stop on your own, ask your doctor for advice on how to put your resolution into practice.

Help is at hand

Learning to love exercise

Does being told to take more exercise make you want to lie on the sofa and cover your ears? Or are you worried that having diabetes will mean you have to give up something you really enjoy? Whatever your reaction, you could be in for a pleasant surprise.

Couch potatoes may need to 'psych' themselves up to doing something active, and it helps to think about the rewards to come as listed here:

- Regular exercise will give a terrific boost to your overall health and sense of well-being. By improving your fitness, you could bring about a drop in blood pressure and in the levels of blood fat – both of which will reduce your risk of heart disease.
- In itself, exercise can help lower blood sugar levels
- When trying to lose weight seems like a battle you'll never win, exercise can be an

Before exercising, you should take some extra carbohydrate, preferably in a form that is absorbed rapidly, e.g. a chocolate bar, sugar lumps or a sweetened high-energy drink. This helps prevent a hypoglycaemic reaction.

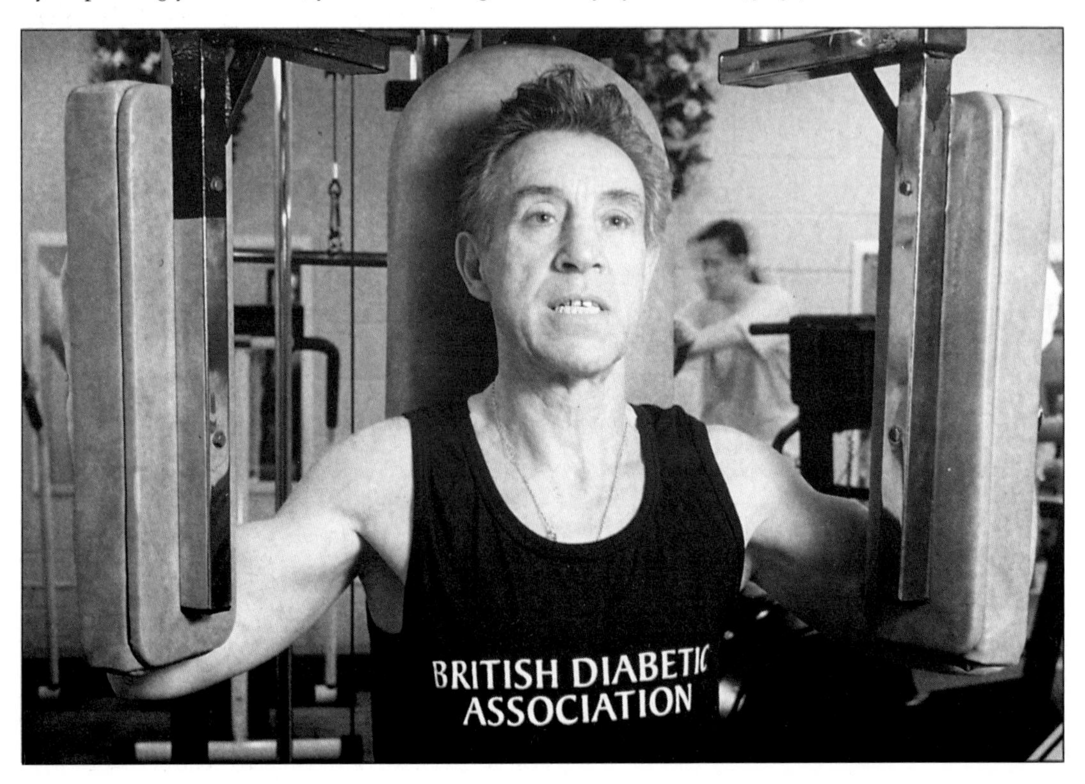

The benefit of exercise

Most people would benefit from taking more exercise – and this is especially true for anyone with diabetes as it can help lower your blood sugar levels. This doesn't mean taking up squash or swimming a mile a day. Just 20 to 30 minutes a day two or three times a week is enough. It's best to start with something relatively gentle like walking if you're not used to it. You will need to plan your exercise programme to balance your food intake, especially if you are on insulin or sulphonylurea tablets to avoid having a hypo (for more on how to do this, see page 44)

important ally. You'll burn up some of those calories and may even improve the rate at which your body burns up energy so you are less inclined to gain weight.

- Everyday events like climbing stairs or carrying heavy shopping will be less of a strain – no more puffing and panting.
- However reluctant you are to begin with, you'll find that a bout of exercise will leave you feeling a glow of self–satisfaction and pleased that you made the effort.
- Don't forget that exercise doesn't have to mean jogging miserably round damp streets or forcing yourself to take part in something you never wanted to do. Dancing or bouncing on a mini–trampoline, for example, are just as worthwhile as squash or sessions on an exercise machine.
- A body that's toned by regular exercise looks much better than one that's sluggish and sagging, even though you might never get super-fit!

Sports enthusiasts know all this already, and the good news for you is that having diabetes is no bar to having fun or even excelling in your chosen field. With advice from your specialist and a bit of experience, you'll soon find out what works best for you.

The Premier League footballer Gary Mabbut is diabetic. However, he has successfully controlled his diabetes and is a shining example to young people of how they can participate and excel in sport in spite of their diabetes.

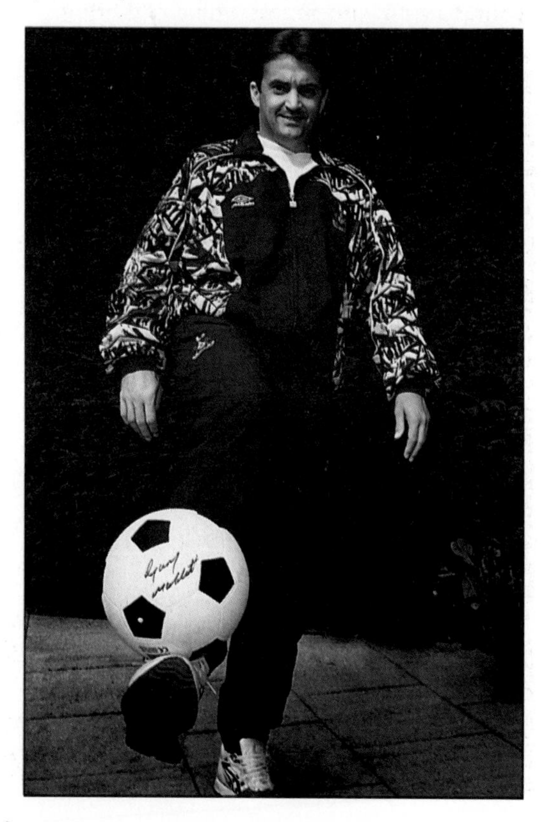

Help is at hand

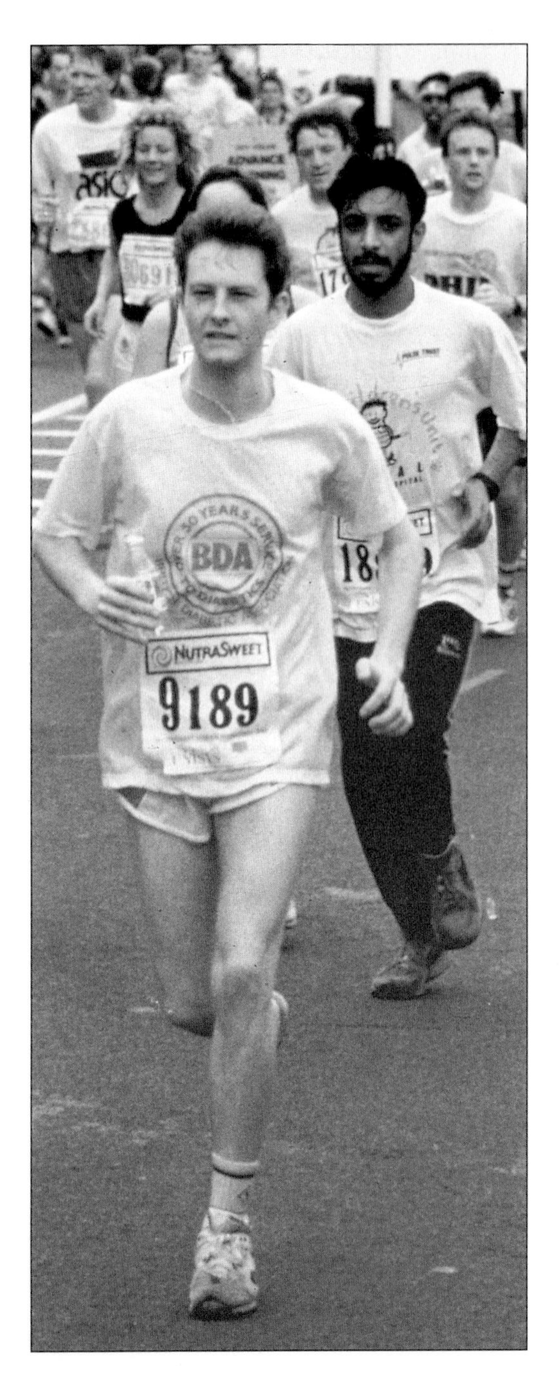

People whose diabetes is treated by diet alone or with metformin tablets need have no worries that exercise will cause problems with their condition, although it may be worth having a general health check–up if you're planning to take up a new type of sport for the first time.

People taking sulphonylureas or insulin need to take precautions against sudden dramatic changes in blood sugar levels which exercise can bring about. You need to be aware that you can end up with too much sugar in your blood because exercise hormones – especially adrenaline – counteract the effects of insulin. Nevertheless, the more important risk is of having a 'hypo' because you are burning up energy and so reducing your blood sugar level. Once you know what the dangers are, you can take the necessary precautions to prevent problems arising.

There are two possible approaches: eating extra carbohydrates before (and possibly after) an exercise session, or reducing your insulin or tablet dose beforehand. Some people find that a combination of both suits them best. With protracted sessions, such as a long run, for instance, you may need to feed on the hoof too.

Talk to your diabetes team about how to plan these adjustments, then measure your

Provided that you take the correct measures before exercising, i.e. taking extra carbohydrate or maybe reducing your insulin dosage if the exercise is particularly strenuous, there is no reason why you should not enjoy such sports as marathon running.

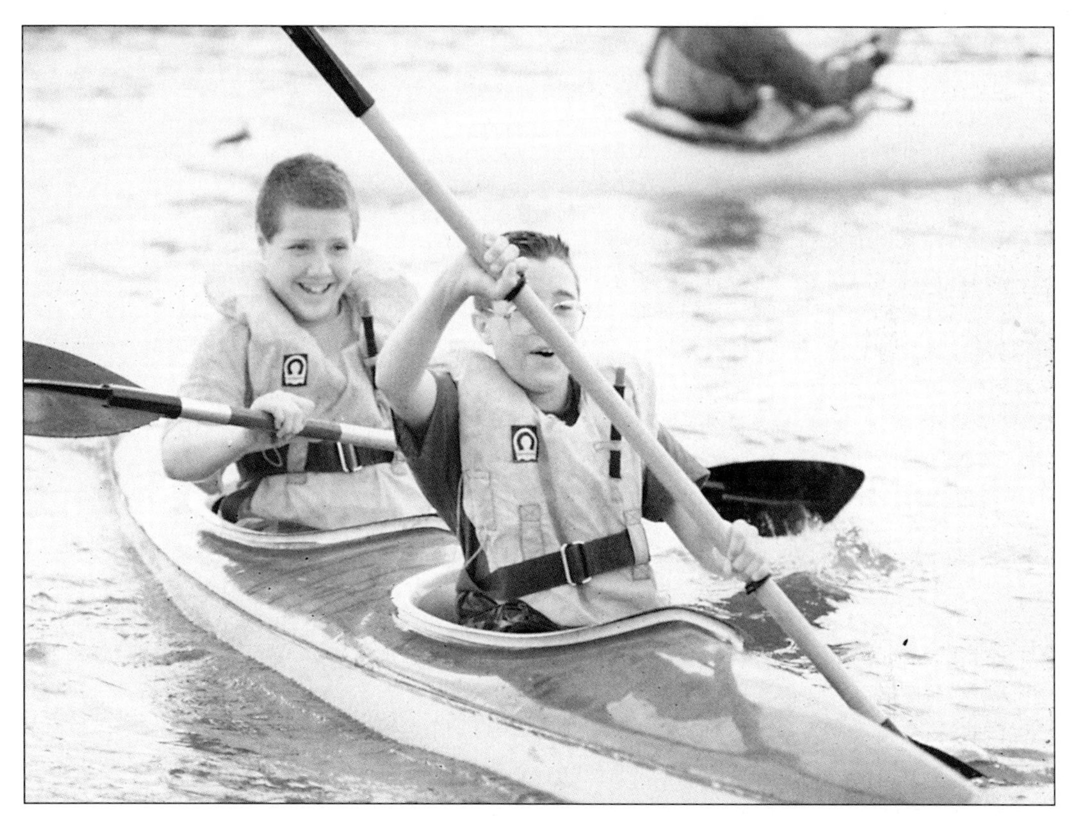

Children should be encouraged to participate in a wide range of sports. However, they should only take part in more hazardous sports such as canoeing or rock-climbing under adult supervision in case they become hypoglycaemic.

blood glucose level before you exercise, and take it several times later in the day too. Some people find they're fine immediately after a session, then have a hypo later on.

How much adjustment you need will vary from one person to another, but will also depend on the type and duration of the exercise. A brisk walk may not require too much extra carbohydrate, while a game of football may mean you'll need more of an energy boost. Work out what you think you'll need as carefully as you can beforehand, but be prepared for a certain amount of trial and error. In case you get it wrong at first, keep a supply of quick–acting carbohydrate, such as a bar of chocolate or a can of Lucozade, where you can get to it immediately if you need to.

When you give yourself an injection before a bout of exercise, the best site to use is your stomach. Injecting in a limb which is going to be using a lot of energy is likely to mean the insulin is absorbed more quickly than usual, increasing the risk of a hypo.

Chapter four

Make it easy on yourself

While there is no reason why your diabetes should limit your options in any important ways, there are times when you will need to take extra care of yourself and plan just a bit more carefully than other people. Any activity or change to your usual routine which has the potential to disrupt your diabetes needs to be thought about, and possibly discussed with your diabetes team, but there is little you can't do with the right kind of advance planning.

Having a baby

Pregnancy places considerable strains on any woman's body – after all, it requires a great effort to grow a new human being! It is essential if you have diabetes to start planning for this well in advance and your first step should be to discuss your plans with your doctor and specialist nurse. In some areas, there are pre-pregnancy clinics where women with diabetes can talk over what they need to do both before and during pregnancy to ensure that they and their babies get through with the minimum of problems.

You will certainly be told that the key to having a relatively trouble-free pregnancy and a healthy baby is very good diabetic control which needs to be established before you conceive. This is likely to mean more frequent blood sugar testing and making fine adjustments to your diet and insulin regimen, with the aim of getting your blood glucose levels as close as possible to normal before meals. It is likely that your carers will take the opportunity at this point to give you a thorough health check to ensure that there are no underlying problems which could make pregnancy difficult or complicated.

Many women find the first few weeks of pregnancy the most difficult, especially if they suffer from morning sickness and find they don't want to eat as well as usual. Obviously, this situation is more serious when you have diabetes, and your dietitian will be able to give you advice on how to cope if you are unlucky enough to suffer from a lot of nausea. It is especially important that you are aware of the increased risk of having a hypo – which is most likely in the first 16 weeks and the last few weeks of pregnancy.

Once your pregnancy is underway, you will be monitored very carefully – for example, you will have more frequent ultrasound scans than someone who hasn't got diabetes, and your doctor will also advise you about the likelihood of your needing more insulin as the

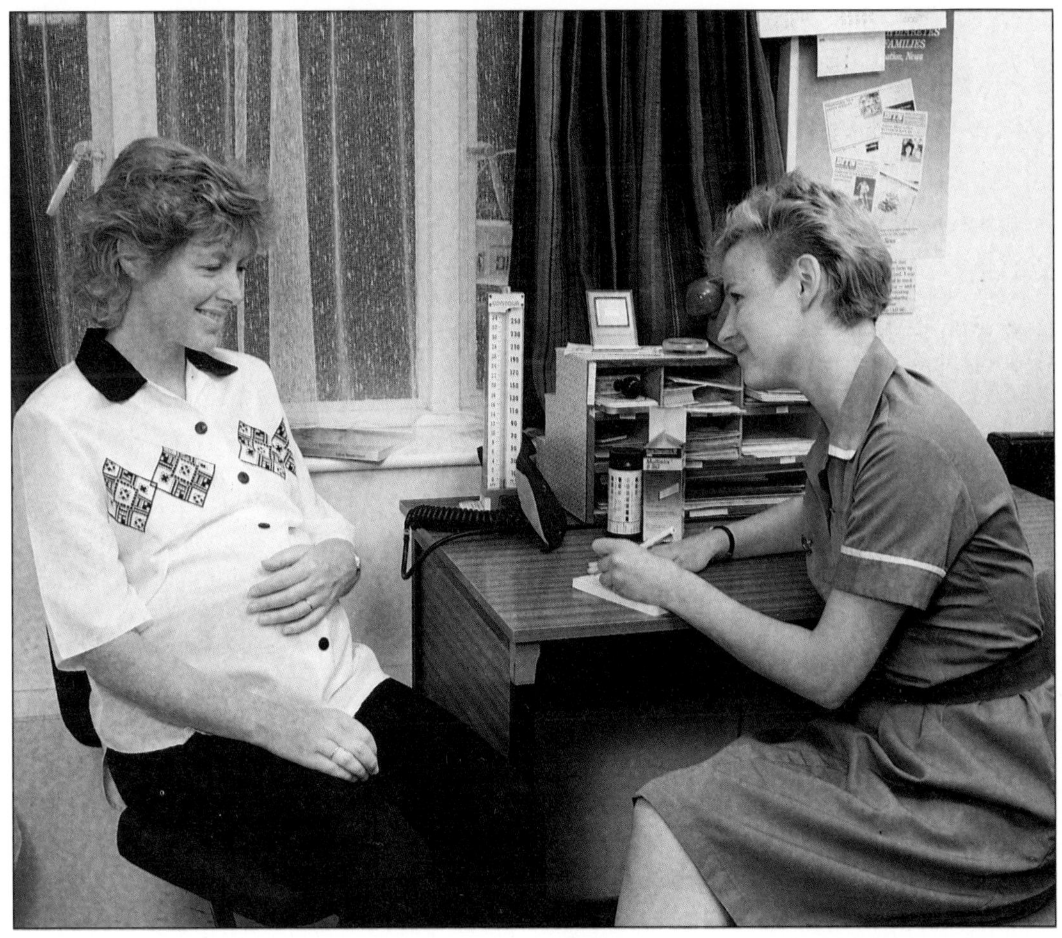

During pregnancy, you must control your diabetes carefully and monitor your condition with either urine tests or blood tests. You may need to liaise closely with your doctor, specialist nurse, midwife and consultant.

months pass. Many women with diabetes give birth naturally these days – although you do have a slightly greater than average chance of a Caesarean delivery – and you won't be allowed to continue past your due date. Induction at around 38 or 39 weeks is common if nature doesn't arrange the baby's arrival before that, and the birth is virtually certain to be in hospital.

Having said all that, there is no reason why a woman with diabetes should not have a healthy pregnancy with a healthy baby at the end of it. The secret is in very good control, which really is an excellent incentive to make the extra effort required to achieve it.

Pregnancy checklist

- Talk to your consultant, specialist nurse, dietician and ideally the obstetrician who will look after you in pregnancy several months before you plan to conceive.
- Work in conjunction with your medical advisers to ensure that your diabetic control is as good as it possibly can be both before and during pregnancy.
- While some 60 per cent of pregnant women don't suffer severe hypos, it's wise to be prepared and make sure your partner, colleagues and others you spend a lot of time with are aware of the possibility and know what to do if necessary.
- If you're feeling tired, make sure you don't accidentally sleep through your normal mealtimes.
- While you can continue with mild exercise, make sure that you check your blood sugar level before you start and adjust your insulin dose or your carbohydrate intake if necessary.
- Find out as much as you can in advance about what will happen at the birth. While you will be connected to various drips, you should still have a choice about pain relief and the position you adopt for the actual delivery. Talk to your midwife about this beforehand so you are well prepared when the big moment arrives.
- Be prepared for the fact that your newborn may be whisked away to special care as soon as he is born to check that all is well. It's nothing to worry about – and he should be back with you very soon.

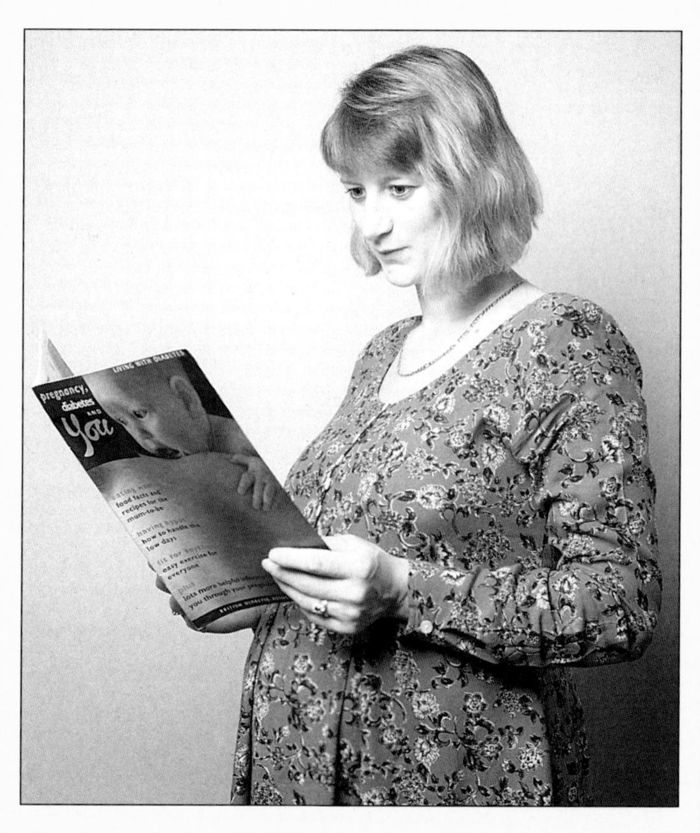

When you're under the weather

Everyone knows that even a relatively minor illness like a bad cold or flu can make you feel really rough, but if you have diabetes as well you must take proper care of yourself. Just having some kind of bug will make your blood glucose rise, even if you're being sick or not up to eating anything much. If you're not aware of the risks, you could quite quickly find that you've got symptoms of uncontrolled diabetes all mixed up with those caused by the illness. The list of infections you need to watch out for includes:

- Common viruses, like colds and flu.
- Chest infections, such as bronchitis.
- Anything which causes diarrhoea and/or vomiting, such as gastroenteritis.
- Urinary infections, such as cystitis.
- Skin infections, such as boils or inflamed cuts and ulcers.

When you're not eating and don't even have an appetite, it may seem pointless to keep taking your tablets or insulin, but stopping is the worst thing you can do. In fact, people with IDDM may even need more insulin than usual, and if you usually take tablets, you may need to go on to insulin for a short while. Ask your diabetes team for guidelines about this before you get ill, and keep them somewhere handy so you can refer to them if the need arises. You'll need to test your blood glucose levels at least four times a day if you aren't already doing so, and you must do this even if you don't much feel like it. Remember that you don't necessarily have to have solid food to keep up your carbohydrate intake; milk, soup and cold drinks like Lucozade or cola can be substituted, but ask your dietitian for advice on the right way to do this if necessary.

Anyone with diabetes who is constantly being sick should get someone to ring the doctor for advice or to ask him to visit. In any case, it's worth consulting your doctor in the early stages of even a mild illness in case there's any treatment you can have to prevent it getting worse. Unfortunately, antibiotics won't help a cold or flu, but they might be worthwhile if you have a bacterial infection.

Remember

- Never stop taking your insulin or tablets even if you are ill or have lost your appetite.
- Always replace your solid food with substitutes if your appetite is poor. Do not be tempted to skip meals. If you are unsure of what to eat, ask your doctor or dietitian for advice.
- Monitor your blood glucose regularly. Test the levels at least four times a day whether you feel like it or not.
- Consult your doctor if you are ill, especially if you are constantly being sick. This may help prevent you getting worse.

Make it easy on yourself

When you're off on holiday

Going away, whether it's in your own country or abroad, is all a matter of confidence and planning. When your destination is somewhere you've never been before, or if it involves a long journey through one or more time zones, it may be useful to talk over any possible problems with your doctor or nurse specialist.

Remember too that you may need immunizations if you're going somewhere really exotic, and you need to plan this well in advance. Your doctor will be able to tell you

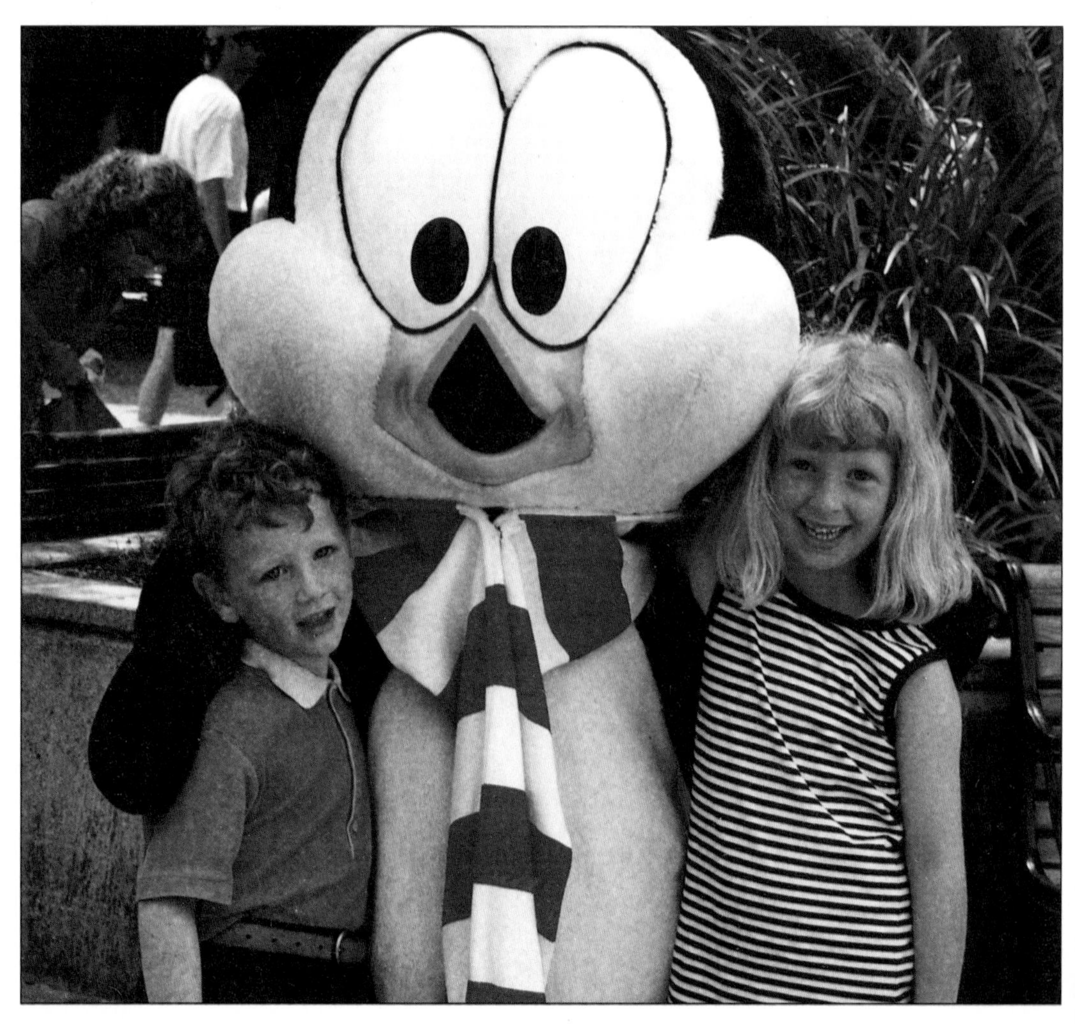

what's needed where you're going, and work out a timetable for your immunizations if necessary. Don't take any chances regarding food either – ask what you should do if the dreaded travellers' tummy strikes. You could be badly affected if you suffer from severe diarrhoea and vomiting, and though it's unlikely, it's as well to be prepared. You might also find it useful to know the carbohydrate content of some of the foods you might be offered instead of your usual potatoes or cereal, for example. Check these out in advance before your departure.

Seasoned travellers will know only too well that a journey of any length rarely goes completely according to plan; hold–ups somewhere along the line may not be inevitable, but it's wisest to assume the worst and prepare for it! At least, it's worth taking supplies of food and drink in your hand luggage, in case the coach breaks down, the plane is delayed or the train has no buffet. Sandwiches made with wholemeal bread, chocolate and fruit make the ideal combination of fast–acting and more slowly absorbed carbohydrates to cover every situation.

Even if you're already adept at packing your medical supplies, it's easy to forget something in the rush of departure if you don't make a checklist.

You shouldn't have any problems with customs abroad when carrying your syringes and medication, but you may like to ask your doctor for a letter on his headed paper explaining that you have diabetes and giving details of your treatment just in case. You should also have an identity card or a bracelet or other wearable item which indicates that you have diabetes. In the UK the BDA can supply an Insulin Users Identity Card, which carries your photo and important information translated into four other languages. It verifies your need

Packing checklist

Before you leave, make sure you have packed in your hand luggage:

- Insulin and syringes or tablets, plus any other medications you take regularly.
- Test strips.
- Lancets and finger–pricking machine.
- Meter and batteries.
- Record book.
- Glycagon kit and glucose tablets.
- Insurance documents .
- Identity card.

Travel precautions

In addition, if you suffer from travel sickness, check with your doctor what medication is safe for you to take. You can also take the following precautions:

- Ensure that your travelling companions know that you have diabetes and what to do in the event of a hypo or other emergency.
- Tell the air crew you have diabetes.
- Remember that due to time zone changes it may be necessary to take your insulin at a different time.
- Check on medical arrangements at your holiday destination.

Make it easy on yourself

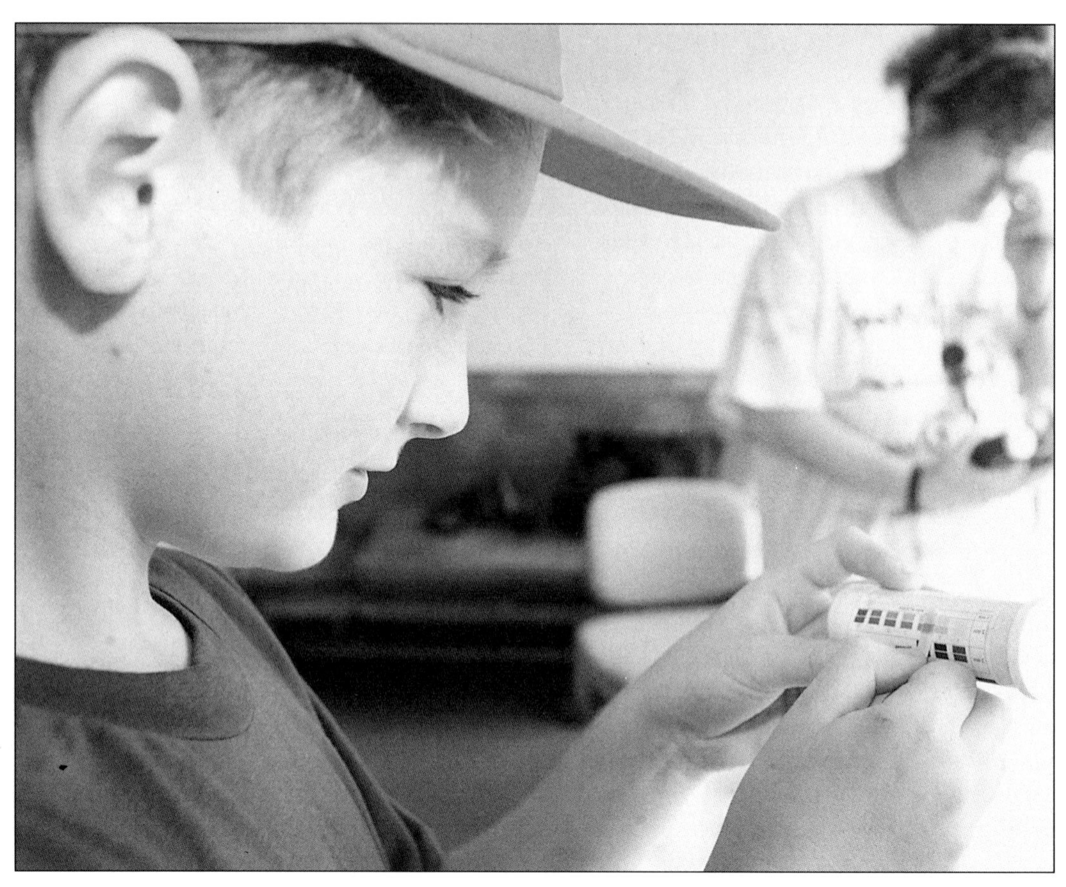

to carry syringes and medical equipment and will help avoid any hassle at foreign customs points.

You are likely to be able to obtain further supplies of insulin, syringes, tablets and testing equipment in most holiday destinations if necessary, although you will need to know both the brand names and the generic names and to check the strength of insulin used in case of any confusion. Again, if you think you may need to obtain further supplies abroad, you can get details of what's available where from the BDA in the UK.

Anyone taking insulin will already know that it should normally be kept in the fridge. However in practice it will not lose its effectiveness if kept for up to a month at room temperature, provided it's not subjected to very hot or cold conditions. This is one reason why you should never pack it in a bag which will go in an aircraft hold as it will freeze. Many people find the easiest way to transport their insulin is in a box made of some insulating material like polystyrene or a wide–necked vacuum flask. Insulin which is normally clear will look cloudy when damaged, while the normally cloudy sort will develop lumps that can be seen when the container is gently turned.

Whatever your normal lifestyle, chances are that you will not be following it too closely while you're on holiday. You may eat different foods at different times, and take more or less exercise than usual. You've probably already worked out that the way to ensure that this doesn't affect your diabetic control is to test your blood glucose frequently so you can correct any fluctuations in level. While it may seem even more of a chore than usual on holiday, it is worth doing so that you can relax and really enjoy your break.

When hypos are a fact of life

People whose diabetes is treated with diet alone or with diet and metformin or acarbose tablets do not have hypoglycaemic episodes, but anyone on another form of treatment will probably experience them sometimes. The first thing to remember is that though embarrassing and alarming at first, they are hardly ever life threatening, and then only when combined with some other serious problem such as alcohol abuse.

Why do hypos happen?

We have already seen how people with diabetes have to adjust their diet, medication and energy consumption to keep their blood glucose levels within normal ranges. When something disrupts this delicate balance, the blood glucose level can drop too low and a hypo will be the result. 'Too low' in this context means below 3 – 4 mmol/l. When this happens, a group of nerves automatically signal that the system has gone wrong, and trigger the release of a hormone called adrenaline to try to correct the situation. Adrenaline will stimulate the release of stored supplies of energy and direct

Symptoms

You may get some or none of these, or some of the ones listed below, but every individual will have a slightly different sensation, which may even change after you have had diabetes for some considerable time.

- Feeling wobbly or shaky
- Feeling very hungry
- Your pulse beats faster than usual or you have heart palpitations
- You start to sweat or feel uncomfortably hot
- Feeling cold
- Tingling around the mouth
- Feeling faint or dizzy
- Blurred vision
- If no action is taken, you will eventually lose consciousness

them to the brain where the need for them is greatest. It is when the nerves send out these 'do something' signals that you may experience the symptoms of a hypo.

Symptoms

You may suffer some of the symptoms listed in the box panel on page 53.Other people may notice that you've gone pale, or have lost concentration, or that you're getting ratty. It's also quite likely that if they venture to suggest that you may be having a hypo and need to take action, you'll deny it fiercely and refuse to do anything about it. Stroppiness is one of the symptoms of a hypo!

A few people may have more unusual symptoms, such as fits, biting their tongue or a temporary paralysis. This doesn't mean that their hypos are more severe or

Do something fast

- Your immediate priority is to boost your blood glucose level quickly – take sugar, honey, a small glass of a sugary drink or a couple of glucose tablets.
- As soon as you feel able, have your next meal if it is due, or if not, a piece of fruit or a starchy snack such as a wholemeal sandwich or a biscuit and a glass of milk. This will prevent your blood glucose level dropping down again once the immediate boost from the sugar or whatever has worn off.
- Obviously, if you lose consciousness before you can take corrective action, you will have to rely on others to deal with the situation. Unless they know exactly what they are doing, they should simply call an ambulance. However this situation is unlikely to arise very often if at all.

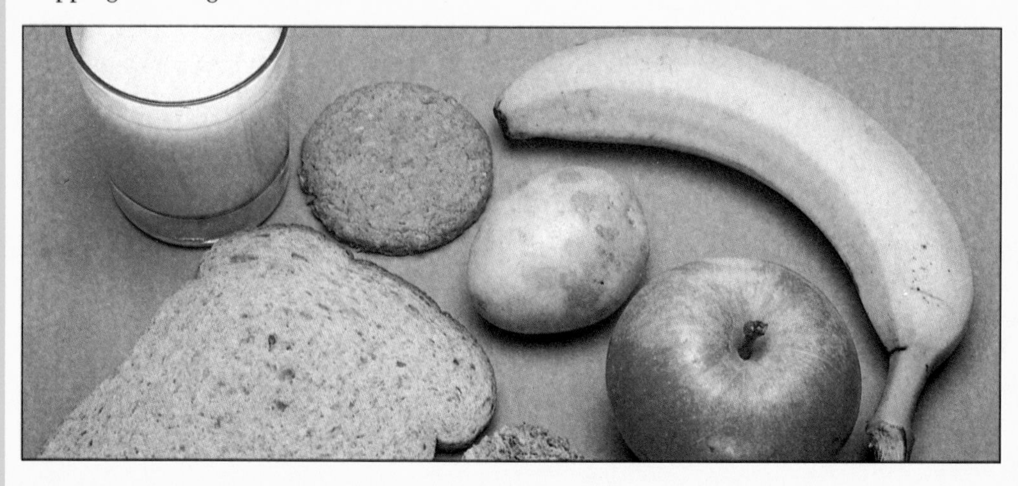

dangerous than anyone else's – just that their symptoms are more dramatic.

A few unfortunate people find that the first thing they know about a hypo episode is waking up with someone mopping their brow and offering them a sugar lump or a sweet drink.No one knows quite why these people don't get warning symptoms or stop having them after a number of years.

Night-time hypos

Many people find they have hypos while they're asleep; around 2 or 3am is quite common. You may wake up, but if you don't, there's nothing you can do at the time! People who do sleep through hypos recover naturally as their liver releases glycogen to counteract the low blood glucose, and wake in the morning feeling tired and hung over, but otherwise unharmed. This is no way to start the day, however, so if this happens to you, you need to do something to stop it. Some people find that a carbohydrate snack last thing before bed does the trick, but otherwise you should discuss the problem with your doctor or nurse specialist as your insulin dose may need adjustment.

What to tell other people

Your immediate family, or some of them at least, will probably have come with you to see the doctor or nurse, so they will be forewarned about what to do if you have a

Checking out the cause

The usual explanation for a hypo is that there has been some upset to the proper balance between food intake, exercise and insulin level. Once you have dealt with the immediate problem, ask yourself what went wrong. The explanation is very likely to be one of the following:

- Missing a snack or a meal, or eating later than you'd planned.
- Unexpected physical exertion, or taking exercise without adjusting your carbohydrate or insulin or tablet dose.
- Accidentally taking too much insulin or getting the timing wrong .

Provided you can pin down what went wrong, you don't need to worry because you'll know how to prevent a repeat performance. However, if there seems to be no reasonable explanation or you have several hypos over a relatively short period, it may be that your insulin regimen needs adjusting, or if you're taking tablets, the type or dosage may need changing. If you're at all unsure, ask your doctor or diabetes nurse. People taking sulphonylureas may experience problems with hypos if they are taking certain other prescribed drugs or sometimes aspirin too. They may also need to be checked for possible liver or kidney problems to make sure these aren't making their treatment less effective.

hypo. However, it does makes sense to talk to any other people with whom you spend a lot of time as well. There's no need to be dramatic or sensational about it, but it would be useful for them to know that there may be times when you need a little help or moral support to deal with an imminent hypo.

Unless they're already well–informed about diabetes, they'll probably be surprised that you could need a very sweet drink or snack sometimes because they probably think having diabetes means you have to avoid sugar altogether. Keep the discussion low key, but explain what you need to do when you are going hypo, and tell them that one of the signs is refusing to recognise the problem and being reluctant to take action.

Although anyone can be taught how to give an unconscious person with diabetes an injection of glycagon which will counteract the insulin or to rub a special sugar gel around their gums, it will probably only be those very close to you who will get involved to this extent. You may need to warn other people though that giving you something sweet to eat or drink is fine while you're conscious, but dangerous if you have already lost consciousness – you won't be able to swallow it. So the best thing for them to do in that situation is phone for an ambulance and tell the paramedics what's wrong when they arrive.

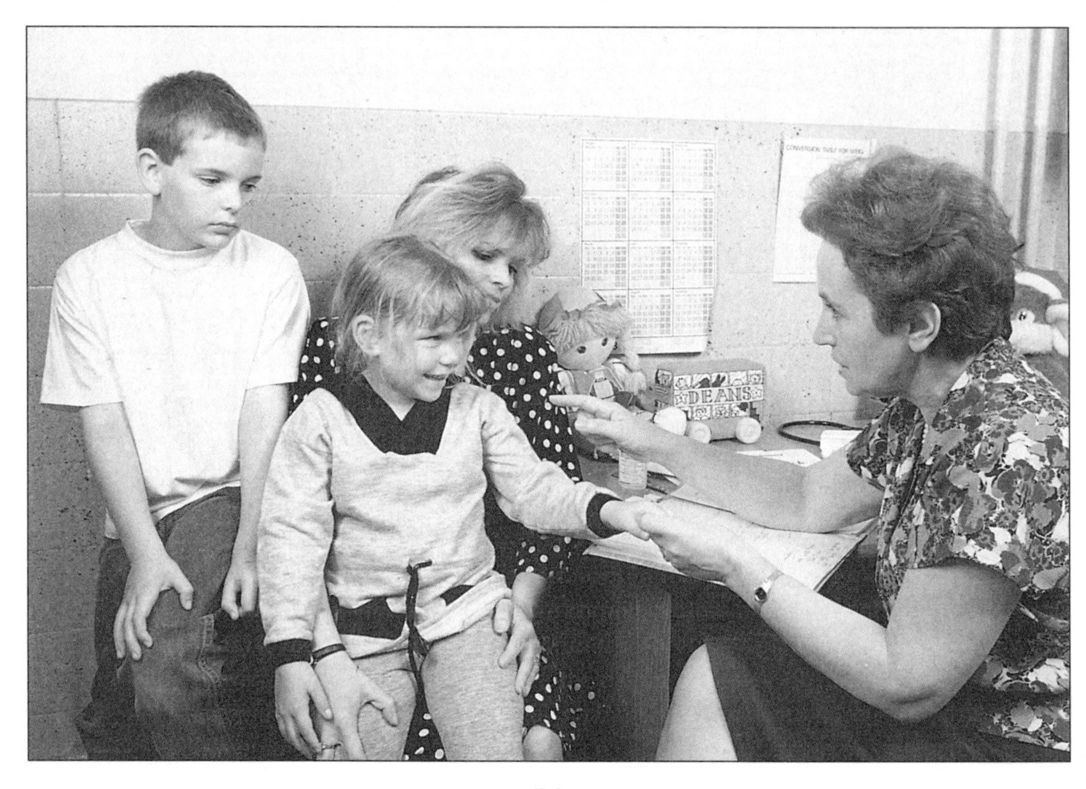

Chapter five

Look after yourself

You already know that as a person with diabetes, you really can't afford to ignore all the self-help advice about looking after your own well-being. A healthy diet, regular exercise, giving up smoking and moderating drinking would make a difference to anyone, but for you they are essential to staying in tip-top health. However, just in case you need any more convincing, there is a long–term effect to be considered.

Although you may think that your condition is hard enough to live with as it is, the truth is that people with diabetes can be prone to developing other health problems. That's the bad news; the good news is that if you succeed in getting your diabetes under tight control and keeping it that way, the risk of developing complications drops dramatically. Only around 15 per cent of people with good control have problems of this kind, as compared to 60 per cent of those whose condition is poorly controlled. And there's more good news: many of the conditions to which you may be susceptible can be warded off by taking a few sensible precautions, while others can be treated successfully if picked up early through regular checks.

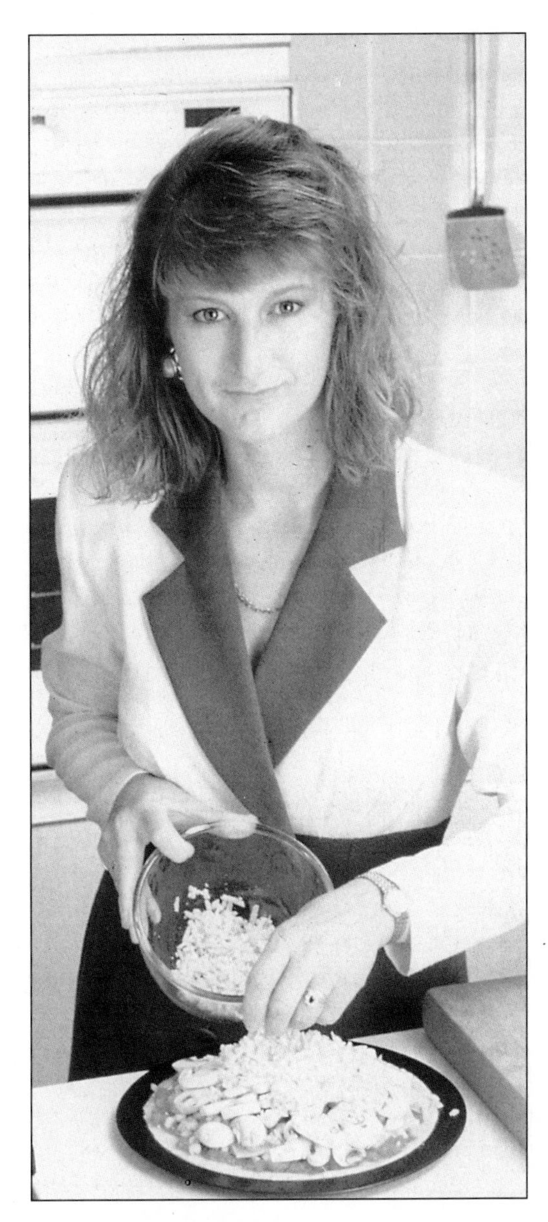

Looking after yourself is very important, and eating regular healthy meals plays an important part in getting your diabetes under control. You can continue to eat a varied diet and enjoy your favourite foods.

Look after yourself

Best foot forward

You may have wondered why a chiropodist featured earlier in the list of people who would help you look after your diabetes. The reason is that diabetes can make the feet susceptible to circulatory problems and nerve damage which can have serious consequences if neglected. However, if you see a chiropodist regularly and follow his or her advice, you will be well on the way to avoiding trouble later.

As with so many aspects of diabetes, much of the advice is straightforward, and applies to everyone. High on the list come

Caring for your feet and inspecting them regularly will help prevent nerve damage later on. Your doctor may suggest that you visit a chiropodist if you have corns, calluses, cracked skin or painful toe nails.

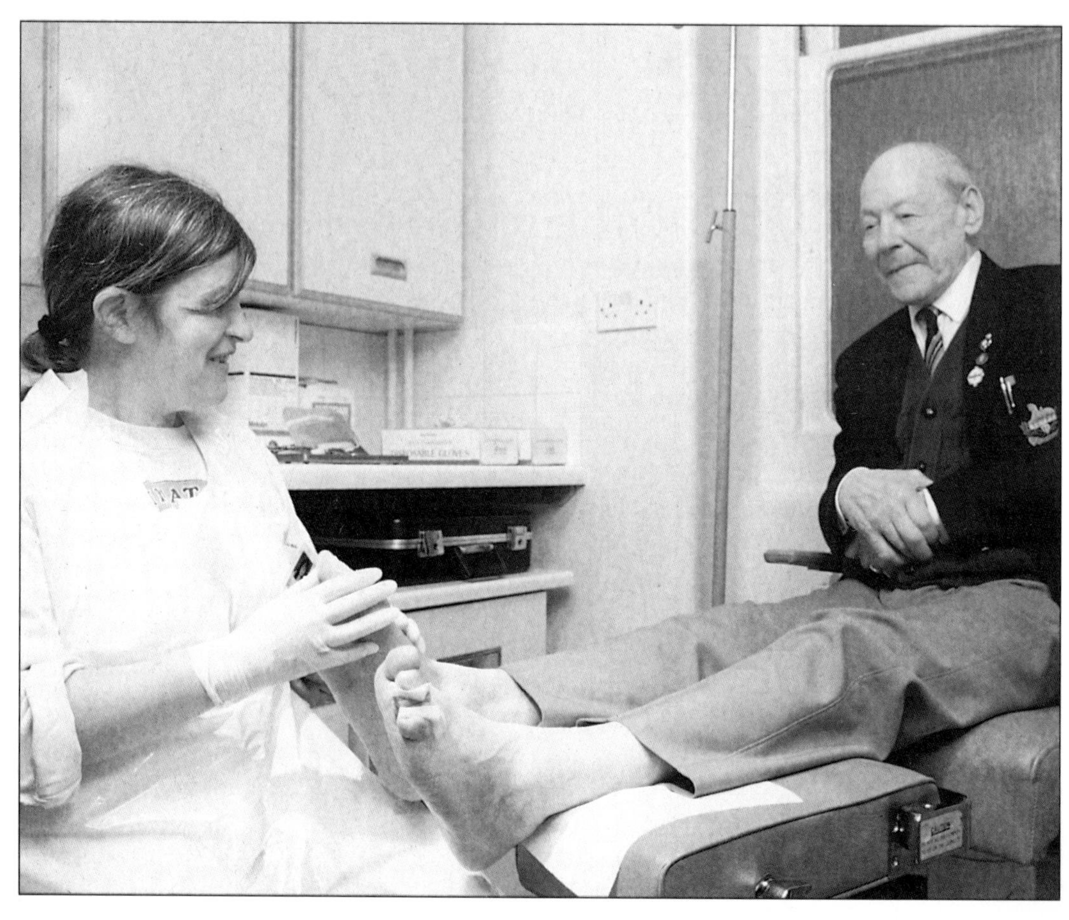

comfortable and well–fitting shoes, giving yourself a regular pedicure and making sure socks and tights fit comfortably and are changed every day. In addition, you will be advised to check your feet daily because minor injuries such as blisters or cuts need prompt first aid if they are not to turn nasty.

People whose non–insulin dependent diabetes was not diagnosed for some time after it began may find they have already developed foot problems such as numb patches, but your doctor or chiropodist can both provide treatment and offer good advice on looking after your feet in the future.

Choosing the right shoes

It is important to choose shoes that are well-fitting, comfortable and provide support. When buying shoes, you should always try them on.

- Your foot should not be able to slide about much inside the shoe.
- There should be adequate room at the front for your toes to move forward naturally as you walk.
- Shoes should feel comfortable immediately; never buy ones that have to be 'broken in'.
- They should be the correct shape for your feet so that your toes are not compressed.

Follow these guidelines and you will take a positive step in preventing diabetic foot problems.

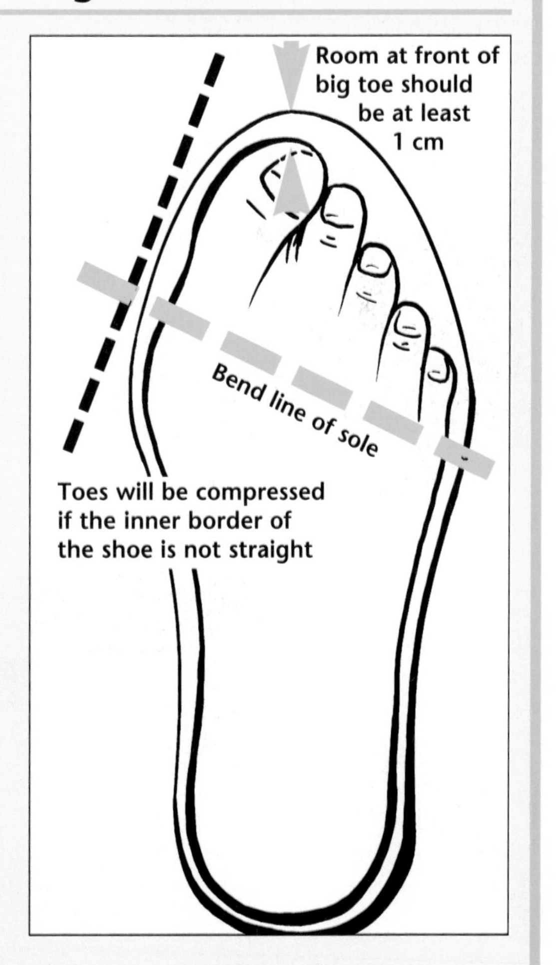

Look after yourself

Eyes right

Many people experience blurring of their vision when they are first diagnosed or as a result of an episode of poor control, but this is only temporary. For others, the first inkling they had that something was wrong was when the optician giving them a regular eye examination suggested they see their doctor. This is because untreated diabetes can cause extra tiny blood vessels to grow at the back of the eye which are visible when the eyes are examined. It can be a shock to be told that you have this problem because you won't have noticed any effect on your eyesight in the early stages.

While it seems that high blood pressure and high blood glucose levels can increase the rate at which this type of eye problem (called retinopathy) develops, good control won't always prevent it happening. However, provided it is picked up in the early stages, retinopathy can very often be treated effectively with the use of a laser. This is why your doctor will recommend that you have your eyes checked once a year.

Staying in good heart

No one is quite sure why diabetes increases the risk of certain kinds of heart disease. The fact that having higher than normal blood glucose leads to a rise in levels of certain types of fat in the blood associated with heart disease may be one factor. Another is that people with diabetes are prone to raised blood pressure, which can make a heart attack (or a stroke) more likely. Whatever the reason, this increased level of risk makes it particularly important to do everything you can to decrease your other risk factors.

Of course, if you manage to follow all the advice you've already been given in connection with your diabetes, you won't have much more to think about. All the following tips are standard advice on reducing the chances of developing heart disease, and you've heard virtually all of them before. Just in case you need reminding, here they are again:

- Give up smoking. It's just about the worst habit to have as far as your general health is concerned, and it's one of the major risk factors in heart disease.
- Lose weight if necessary. Not only will it make controlling your diabetes easier, but it will reduce the strain on your heart. Ask your dietitian for advice on how to do it safely if you're in doubt.
- Watch your blood pressure. Your doctor will check it regularly anyway, but don't ignore his advice if he says yours is too high. He may want you to reduce animal fats and dairy produce in your diet still further and increase your fibre intake, or you may need treatment with tablets. Just because high blood pressure doesn't make you feel bad, it

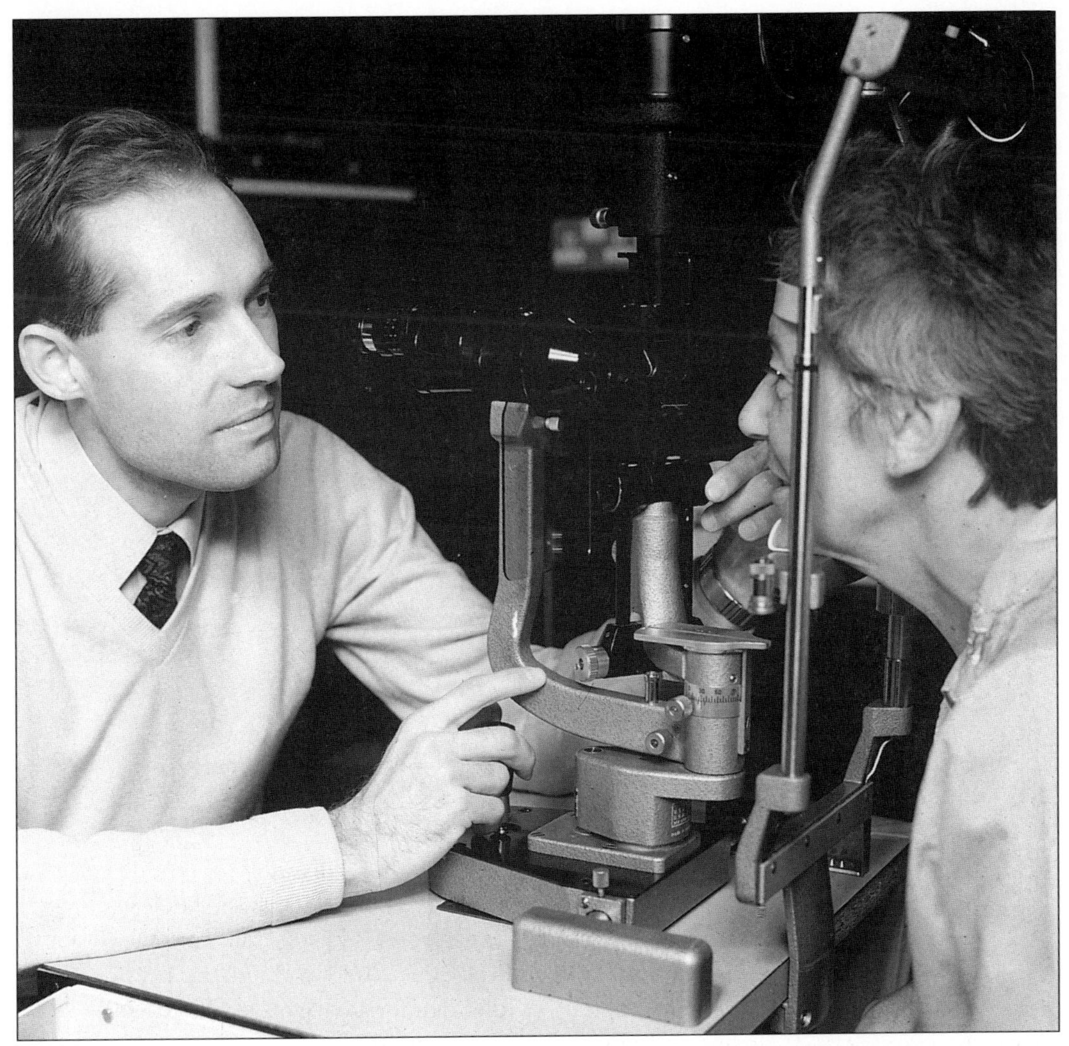

Regular eye checks, will help identify any eye problems before they become serious.

doesn't mean you can afford to ignore it.

- Keep tight control of your blood glucose levels. You are probably doing your best to achieve this already, but if you're backsliding, here's another good reason to try harder.
- Don't be a couch potato. If you've read this far without taking in the benefits of exercise, you haven't been concentrating. Turn back to the section on exercise on page 42 and make up your mind that you really will start to be more active. You might even find you enjoy it!

Losing weight with diabetes

If you are overweight and have diabetes, you will benefit from losing weight in several ways:

- You will be able to control your diabetes more effectively.
- You will feel healthier and fitter.
- You will reduce the risk of developing heart disease.

Adopting a healthier way of eating and your doctor's and dietitian's recommendations will help you to lose weight, but you should not embark on a weight-reducing diet without consulting your doctor and planning it carefully together. It is vital that you control your calorie and carbohydrate reduction carefully or you may get a hypoglycaemic reaction.

Dieting is more difficult when you are taking insulin because it can interfere with your blood glucose levels. It is important to keep your calorie intake steady as fluctuations in calorie intake can also affect the way in which you control your diabetes. Although at least half of your calorie intake will come from starchy carbohydrate foods, because these are high in fibre they will help prevent you putting on weight. High-fibre foods are:

- Whole-grain cereals.
- Wholemeal bread.
- Brown rice.
- Wholemeal pasta.
- Jacket potatoes.
- Beans and lentils.

Reducing your fat intake

Your dietitian will probably recommend that you eat less fat. This will help you to lose weight or, at least, to stabilize your weight. The most obvious ways to do this are by cutting down on the amount of red meat you eat, reducing your consumption of high-fat dairy foods like whole milk, cream, full-fat cheese and butter, and changing to healthier cooking methods, e.g. grilling or steaming food in preference to frying.

You will soon get used to using skimmed milk in your tea and coffee, on your cereal and in cooking. You will even probably prefer it to whole milk eventually. Try to reserve cream for very special occasions and use low-fat yogurt or fromage frais instead.

Eating less sugar

By doing this, you will also be eating more healthily and controlling your weight better. You can sweeten hot drinks and many desserts with artificial sweeteners. Opt for low-calorie soft drinks which have little or no sugar. Avoid sugary biscuits, cakes, sweets, chocolate, golden syrup, buns, pastries, jams and marmalade made with sugar and canned fruit in syrup. There are low-sugar alternatives to most of these foods so that you can still enjoy them. You should only eat the high-sugar versions in emergencies or if you are ill.

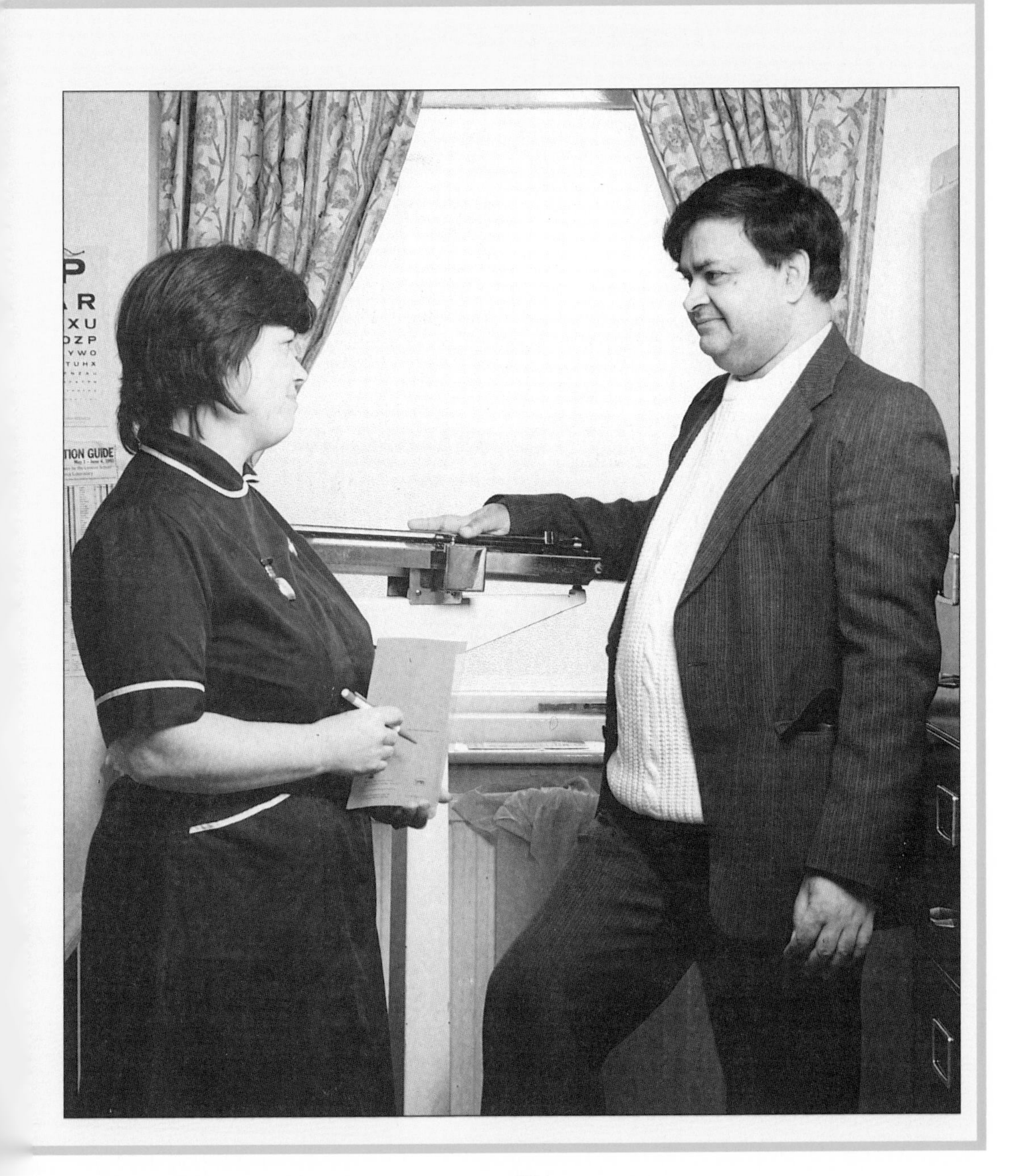
P
R
XU
ZP
YWO
TUHX
TION GUIDE

Exercise your options

Regular exercise will help you to stay healthy and fit as well as improving your well-being and adding another dimension to your life. Just because you have diabetes does not mean that you cannot enjoy and participate in sport. in fact, exercise is good for you and your diabetes. It burns up calories, lowers your blood sugar levels and makes the insulin you take work more effectively, thereby requiring you to take less insulin before exercise.

It is important to take some basic preventive measures before you exercise so that it is beneficial and does not interfere with your diabetes control. If you are planning to exercise, you may find that you can reduce your normal insulin dose before exercising. However, if the exercise is unplanned and you have taken your regular insulin dose, you may need to have a sweet carbohydrate snack before exercising. This will be quickly absorbed into the bloodstream and will counter a fall in blood sugar.

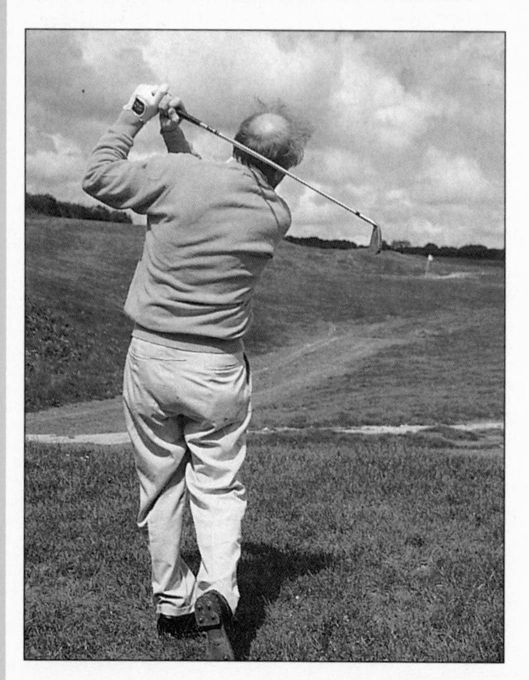

Which sport?

You can do virtually any sport or activity, no matter how strenuous or dangerous. People with diabetes have competed successfully at a high level in a wide range of activities from athletics and marathon running to swimming, football and tennis. It just depends on what you enjoy doing.

Remember that the more strenuous the sport, the more sugar you will use, and you will have to take more carbohydrate or reduce your insulin dose accordingly. Ask your doctor for advice on this. If the exercise is prolonged and performed on a regular basis, then you may need to take less insulin regularly. This is often the case with professional sportsmen and women, and athletes.

Some sports require you to take special care and precautions, especially those which may leave you exhausted, e.g. marathon running, and high-risk activities

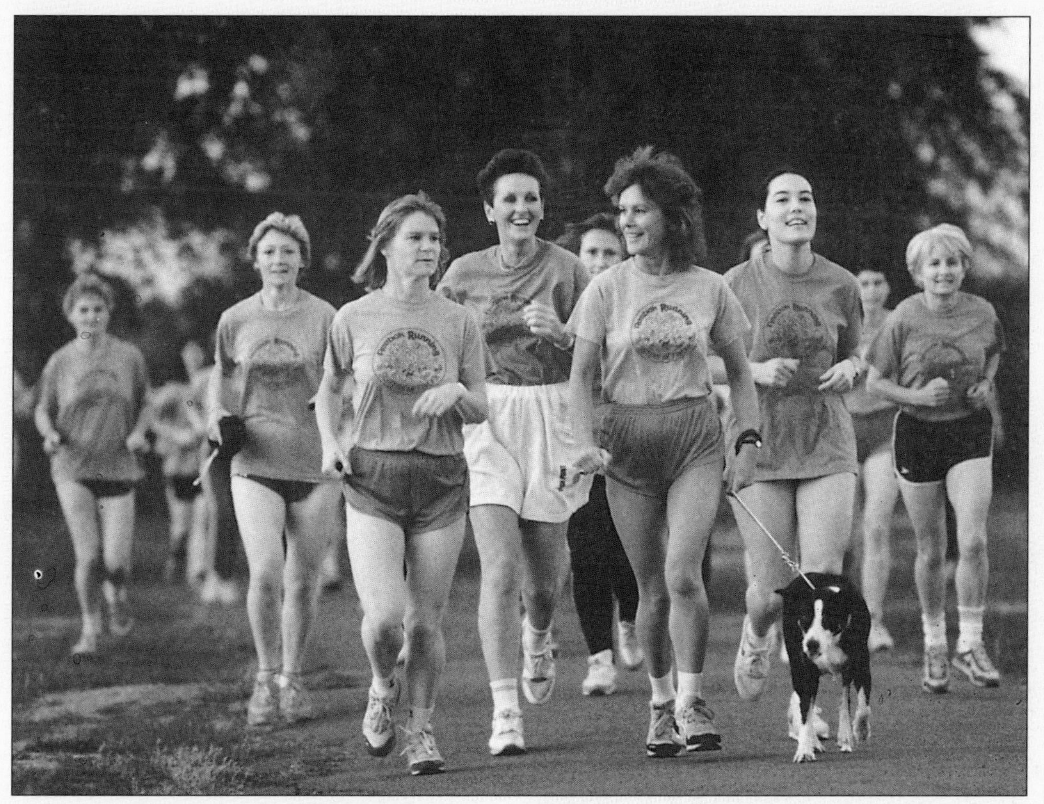

such as rock climbing and hang-gliding. Activities that you do alone without companions or supervision also carry risks, e.g. solo sailing or even swimming. Here are some easy guidelines for you to follow:

- Before you exercise, measure your blood glucose levels.
- Try not to exercise alone.
- If you are accompanied, make sure that your companion knows how to treat a hypo.
- Have a snack before you exercise.
- Take some glucose sweets or sugar lumps with you in case of emergencies.

Remember that hypos are not dangerous in themselves, but they can be potentially dangerous if they happen on the side of a rock face or in a swimming pool. The benefits of regular exercise outweigh these risks as long as you take the necessary precautions.

Chapter six

Practicalities

You may think that it is entirely your own business whom you choose to tell that you have diabetes, but in fact there are a few exceptions to this commonsense rule.

Your working world

As far as work is concerned, you would be unwise to keep your diabetes a secret if there is any chance that your condition may have consequences affecting your efficiency or your colleagues. Many jobs involve shift work, long hours or unpredictable mealtimes, and other people at work will be far more understanding of any problems these factors

Although diabetics can do most jobs perfectly well, there are some that they are precluded from doing, such as the fire service in the UK.

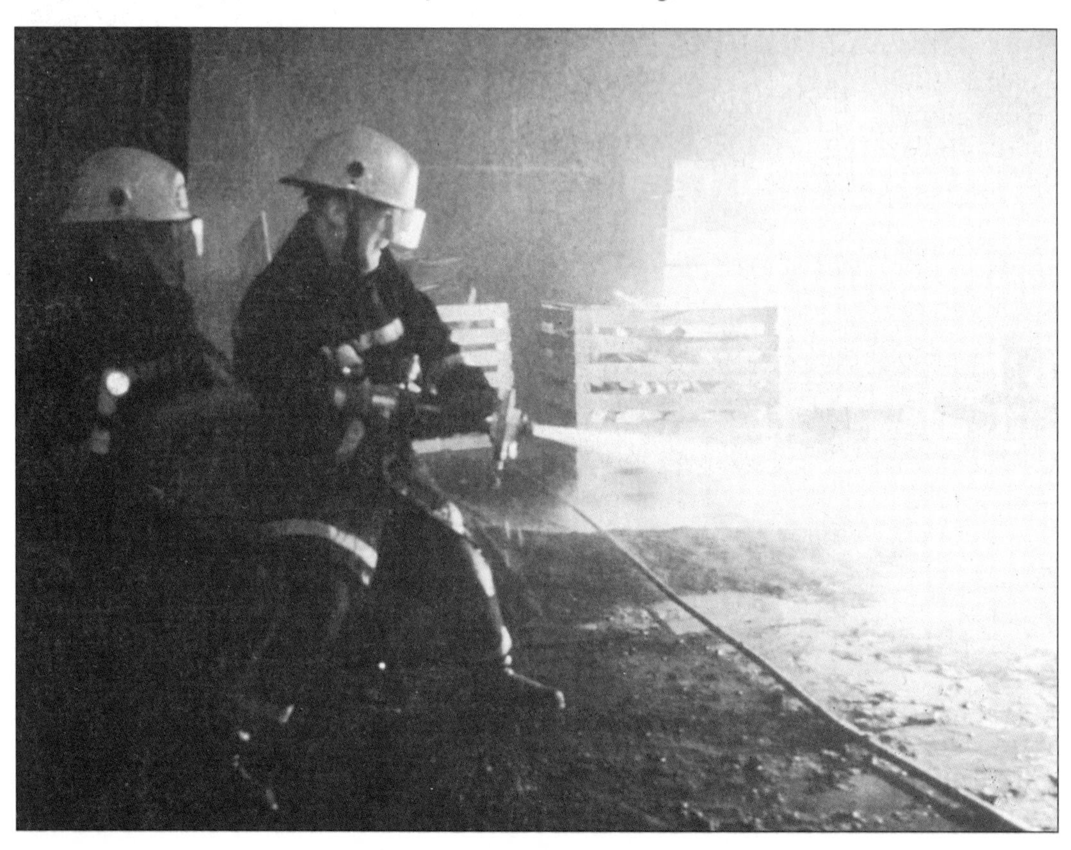

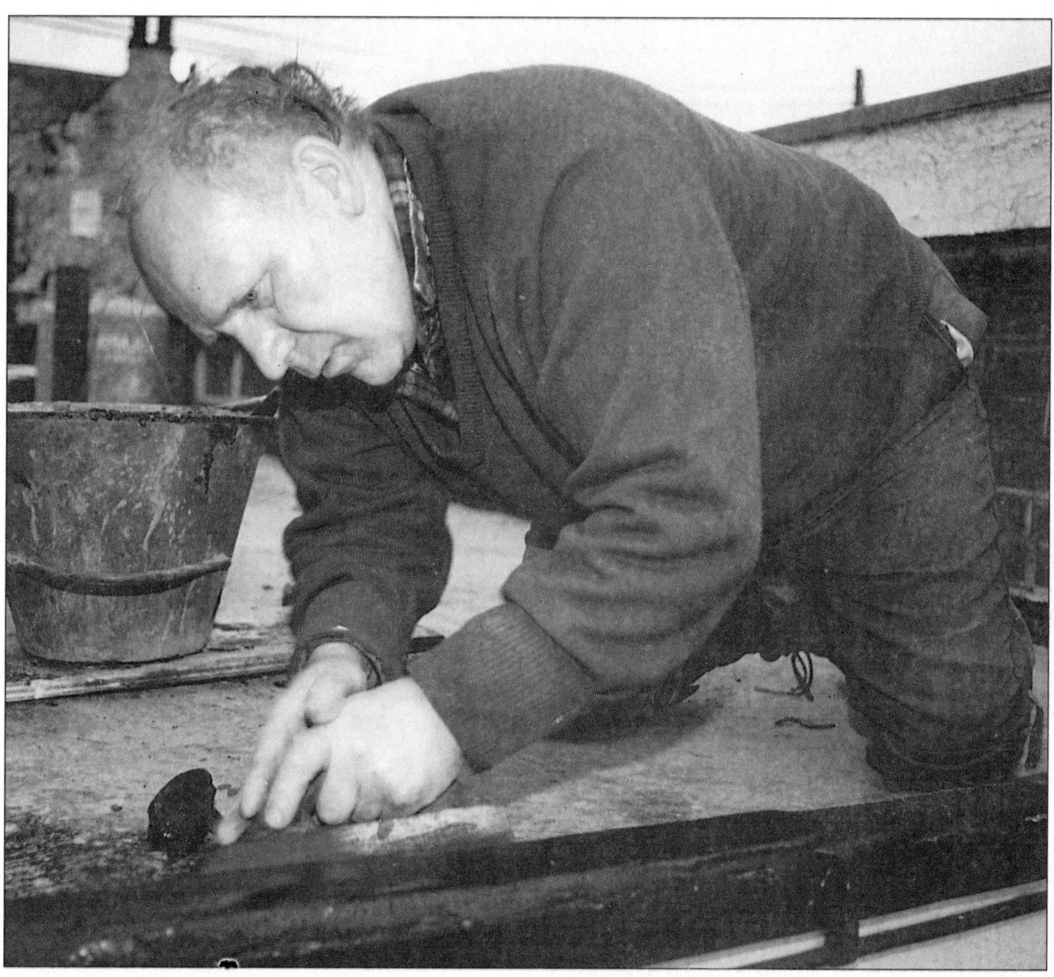

may cause you if they know the reason.

From a health point of view, you may well have no choice about telling the truth if you are at risk of hypos. For example, if your work involves some driving or operating machinery, you could be putting your own safety or that of colleagues at risk if you don't tell anyone.

There are quite a few occupations which simply won't take you on if you have diabetes; in the UK, they range from the police, the armed forces, the fire and prison services to air traffic control, bus driving and the diplomatic service! Of course, if you're already employed in one of these areas, you may be able to stay on, although you might have to move to a different type of work within the organisation. If you live in the UK and have any problems involving employment, you can contact the BDA for advice and support.

Practicalities

On the road

Drivers in the UK are obliged to tell their motor insurance company that they have diabetes. Those who are treated with insulin or tablets must also tell the DVLA (who issue your driving licence), but if you are treated by diet alone, you don't have to inform them unless you develop eye problems which affect your visual acuity or visual fields. If your treatment consists of tablets and healthy eating, you will be issued with a licence that covers you until the age of 70, although you must let the DVLA know if you develop the eye problems mentioned above. People in both these groups should inform the DVLA if their treatment changes; those

Before you set out on a journey in your car, it is a good idea to test your blood glucose level. You can do this easily with a finger-pricking device and handy blood glucose meter.

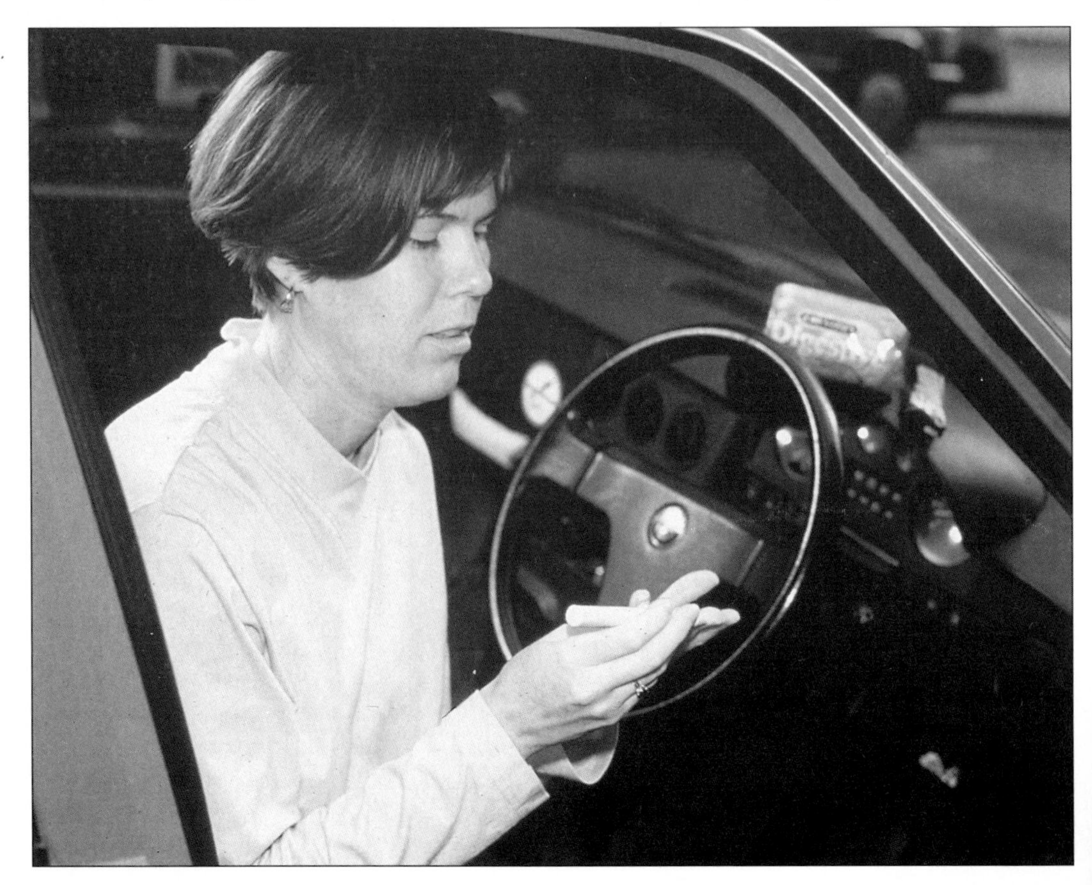

on tablets should let them know if they have to take insulin at any time. Drivers who are treated with insulin will be given a restricted licence that will have to be renewed every one, two or three years, depending on individual circumstances.

There are more restrictions on those who hold a Group II licence, which includes HGV (heavy goods vehicle). As far as those on dietary treatment alone or dietary treatment plus tablets are concerned, the situation is much the same as for ordinary licence holders. However, if you develop visual problems, you must tell the DVLA, who may either withdraw the licence or issue one for a limited period. If you change to insulin treatment, your licence will be revoked, and you won't be given an HGV licence at all if you apply for the first time while taking insulin.

Anyone with IDDM who's had an HGV licence since before April 1991 will have their situation assessed on an individual basis, and annual renewal will be dependent on a satisfactory certificate being provided each year by their consultant.

Insurance companies vary in the way they regard diabetes: some will load your premiums, others won't, and a few seem to make quite arbitrary decisions as to whether they will insure you or not. Some require a lot of tedious form–filling, either by you or your doctor or both. If you have any problems, consult the BDA, who have a specialist insurance broker who can arrange insurance for you.

Hypos are the main potential problem for drivers, and you and your passengers should know what to do if you have one. It's a good idea to do a blood glucose test before you set out on any journey. Once you're on your way, too, you need to be super-alert for the first signs, and keep the necessary supplies of glucose and carbohydrate food with you in case. Don't be tempted to push on just a bit further towards your destination if you know it is really time for you to eat, and allow for the possibility of breakdowns, traffic jams and other delays when working out your journey timetable.

Just in case

There may be times, just possibly, when it is important for other people to know that you have diabetes when you are in no position to tell them. If you are in an accident, unconscious from a hypo or even suffering from keto–acidosis or in a coma because your blood glucose has soared, this knowledge could be vital. The BDA can supply identity cards to keep in your handbag or wallet giving the necessary details. Alternatively, a number of companies make bracelets or necklaces with the relevant details engraved on them. And, of course, there's nothing to stop you buying an ordinary bracelet or necklace and having it engraved yourself.

Whichever option you choose, you should make some clear form of identification a priority. You may never need it, but it's as well to be prepared.

Chapter seven

Question time

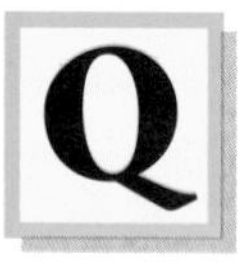

With regular prescriptions and all the kit I need for testing my blood glucose, won't my diabetes cost me a fortune?

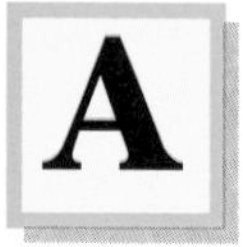

In the UK anyone whose diabetes is treated with tablets or insulin is exempt from prescription charges – you can get an application form from your doctor's surgery. Lancets and strips for testing blood sugar or urine can be prescribed, but if you want a finger-pricking gadget or a blood glucose meter, you will have to buy them. Diabetes magazines carry lots of ads for these products. People whose diabetes is treated by diet alone are not exempt.

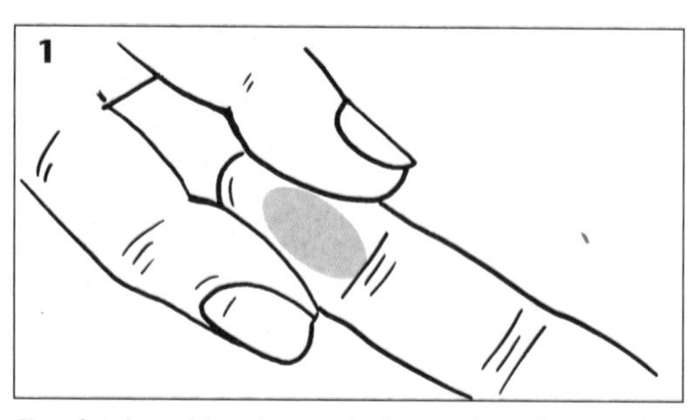

To obtain a blood sample for testing, first make sure that your hands are really clean. Wash them thoroughly. Choose an area on the side of the finger and squeeze until pink (1), then prick with the device to obtain a drop of blood (2). Let it fall onto the testing strip (3), and then follow the manufacturer's instructions.

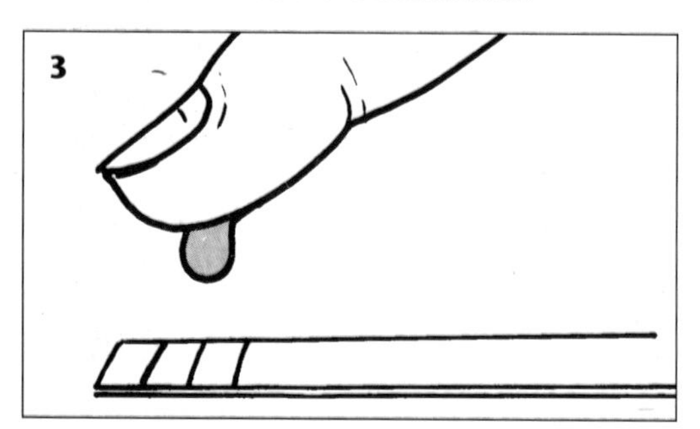

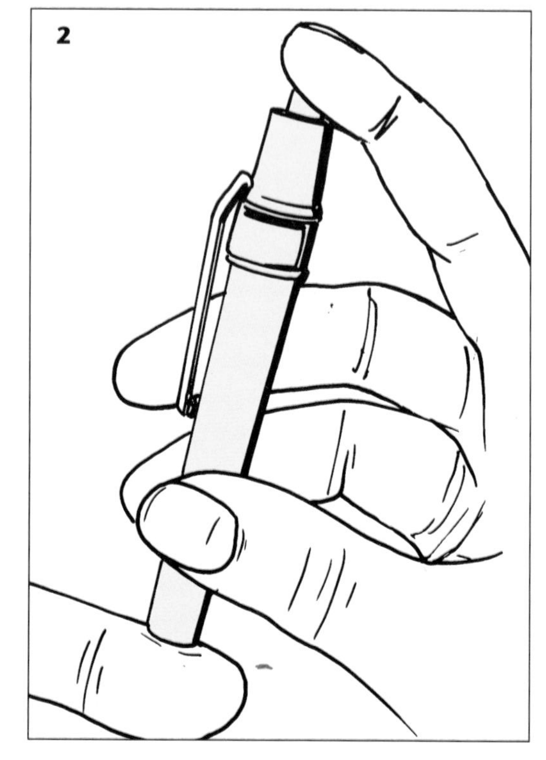

I find fiddling around with syringes and vials of insulin a nuisance; is there an alternative?

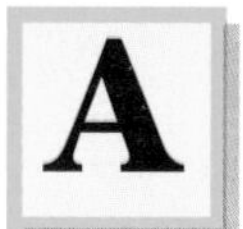

Ask your doctor or specialist nurse to show you the pen devices available. They are pre–loaded injecting devices with a dial you set to determine the insulin dose. You can use one of these if you need several injections a day, or for twice daily injections. Insulin cartridges to use with the pen are available on prescription, and you can also get pre–loaded disposable pens. However, you have to buy the needles to be used with these 'free' pens; your doctor or specialist nurse can give you all the information you need.

Pre-loaded pens

There is a wide range of pen injectors from which you can choose. They are convenient and reliable and are becoming increasingly sophisticated. They have many advantages, particularly their portability. You can keep one in the office at work, in your sportsbag or handbag. You can even carry them in a jacket pocket. Because they are preloaded, they administer an accurate dose of insulin and once the supply is exhausted, you just throw the pen away.

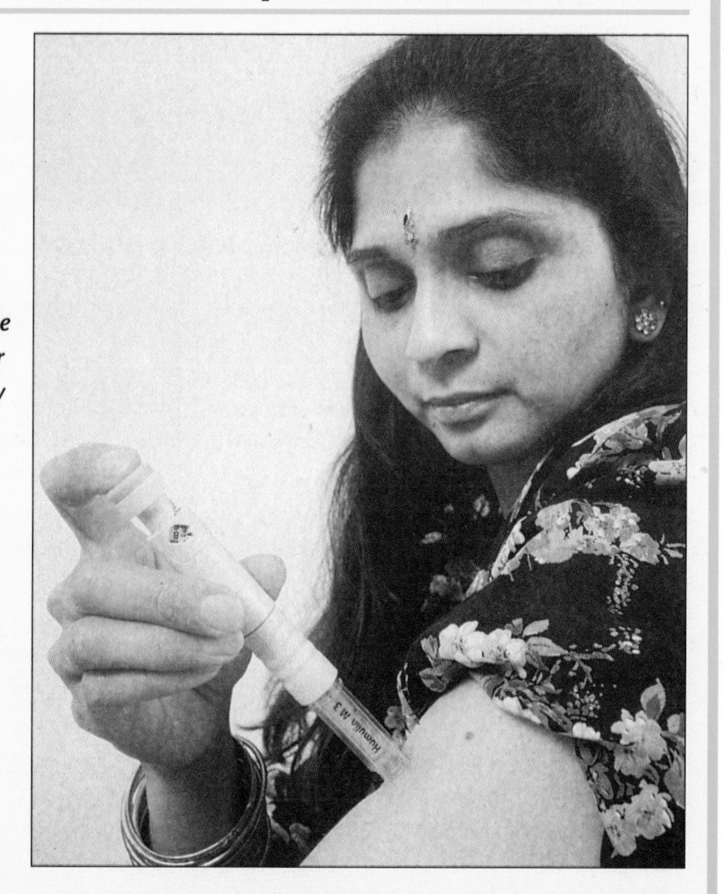

Question time

My doctor wants me to do ketone testing but I don't understand the reason. Why isn't testing my blood enough?

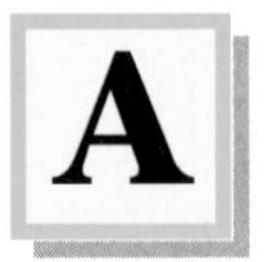

When your diabetes is not well controlled – when you're ill, for example – your blood glucose level may rise, and eventually your body will start to break down fat stores for conversion into energy. One of the by-products of this process is acids called ketones, which appear in the urine. If the build-up is allowed to continue, you could go into a diabetic coma which is obviously dangerous. Measuring your urine for ketones using strip tests will let you know whether this is happening. Ask someone in your diabetes team to go through the reasons why you have been asked to do this test, and make sure you know what to do if you do find ketones in your urine.

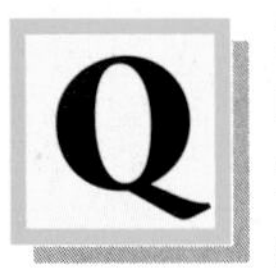

I have heard that people who use human rather than animal insulin don't get any warning signs of a hypo. As I've just started taking insulin, should I ask my doctor to change to animal insulin?

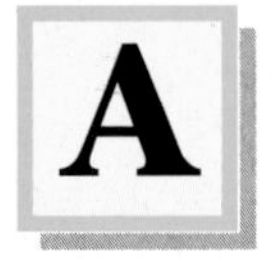

There certainly have been reports that some people who have changed from animal to human insulin found their warning signs changed or disappeared completely. One of the difficulties is that it only happens to some people, and in any case, these changes used to affect some individuals for other reasons, even before the introduction of human insulin. No one is sure why human insulin may affect hypo warnings, although research is currently investigating possible causes. As you have only just started taking insulin, you should not worry. It is likely that you won't experience any problem as only a minority of people with IDDM are affected. If difficulties of this kind do arise, adjustments to your insulin regimen may well solve them. In the last resort, animal insulins are still available for anyone who needs them.

I've been told I've got non–insulin dependent diabetes, but my doctor still insists I do lots of blood tests and take tablets as well as changing my diet. Surely this isn't really necessary as I've only got a mild form of the condition?

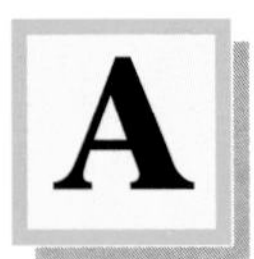

There is no such thing as "mild diabetes". While your type of diabetes seems less dramatic because you don't need injections and because it doesn't come on so suddenly as IDDM, it is still a serious condition which must be treated with due respect. Apart from the fact that you won't feel well if your diabetes is not properly controlled, you will also be much more likely to develop serious complications, such as eye damage and circulatory problems. It may seem like a lot of bother at first, but most people find that it all gets easier with practice, and you'll feel so much better when your diabetes is under control.

Chapter eight

Looking to the future

The two major goals of all researchers working on diabetes are prevention and cure. According to Professor Harry Keen, Chairman of the Executive Council of the British Diabetic Association, progress in the field of prevention is more likely to offer real benefits in the foreseeable future. He is particularly hopeful that it may one day be possible to stop or reverse the process of destruction of insulin–producing cells in the pancreas which ultimately lead to the symptoms of NIDDMM.

At the moment, the body immune response which causes the cell destruction can only be halted by suppressing the response entirely, but ultimately it may be

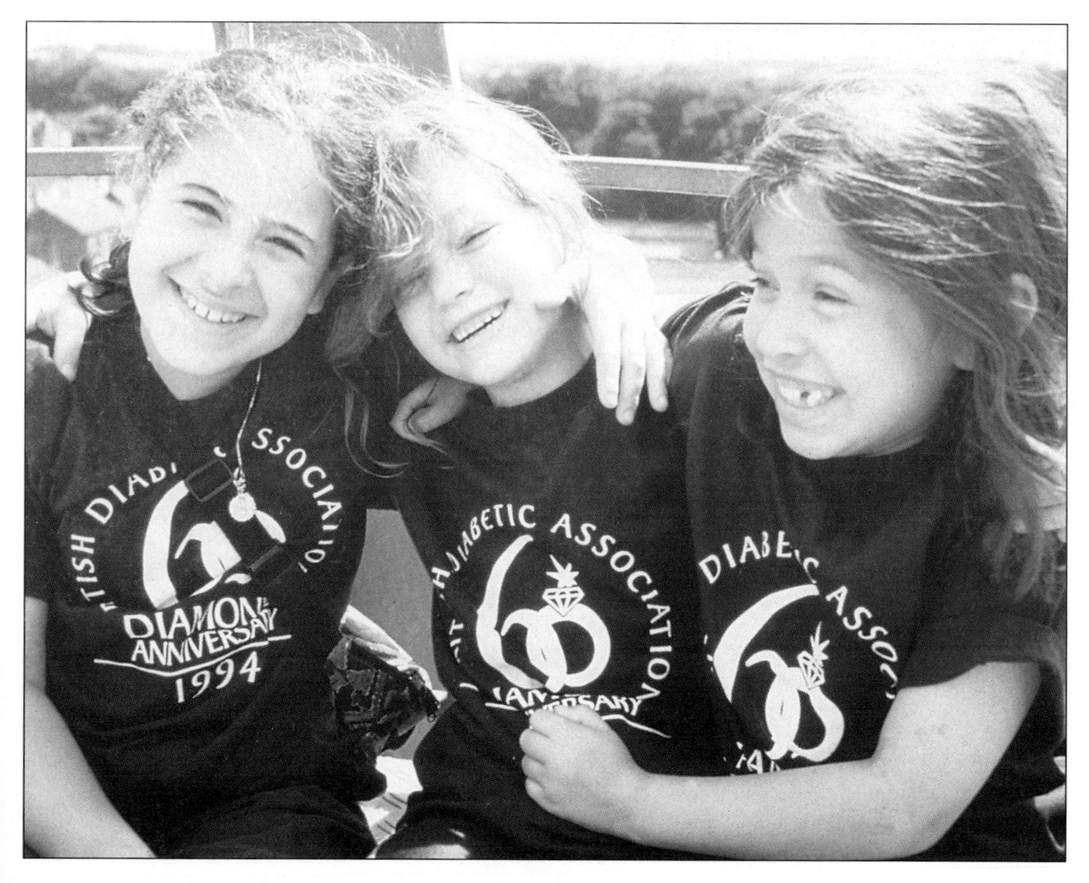

possible to target the specific part of the process which affects the insulin–producing cells. This work he describes as "the eye of the storm" in research terms and one which should lead to practical applications within the next decade.

Although diabetes is known to have a genetic component in some people, developing a screening process which could pick up those who are susceptible is still problematic. Even if it were possible to test all those with a close relative suffering from IDDM, Professor Keen believes this would probably only identify between 10 and 20 per cent of those who will actually go on to develop it themselves. As far as NIDDMM is concerned, attempts to isolate a genetic factor seem to face almost insuperable problems. "It involves such a ragbag of many mechanisms," he points out. "While there may be some people in whom genetic abnormalities play a role, they are only a minority. The possibility of a single gene effect being identified seems

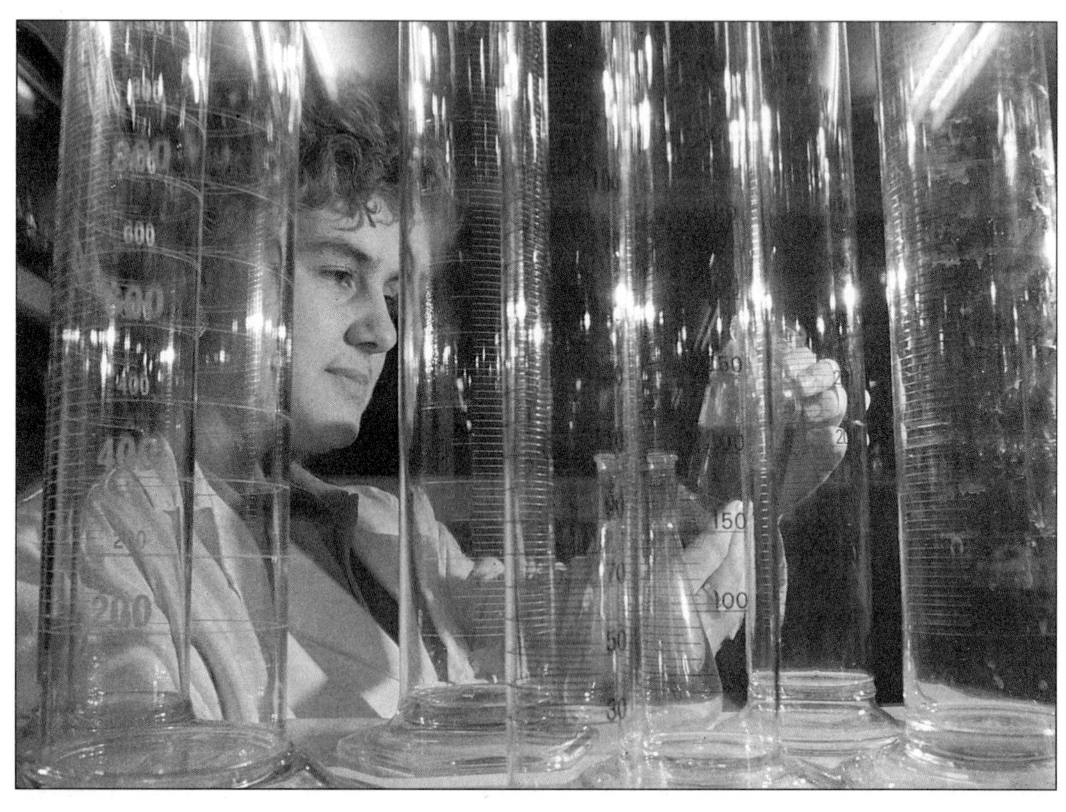

A great deal of research is being carried out to find ways of preventing and curing diabetes, and improving its treatment and reducing complications. The British Diabetic Association in the UK plays an important role in funding this important research.

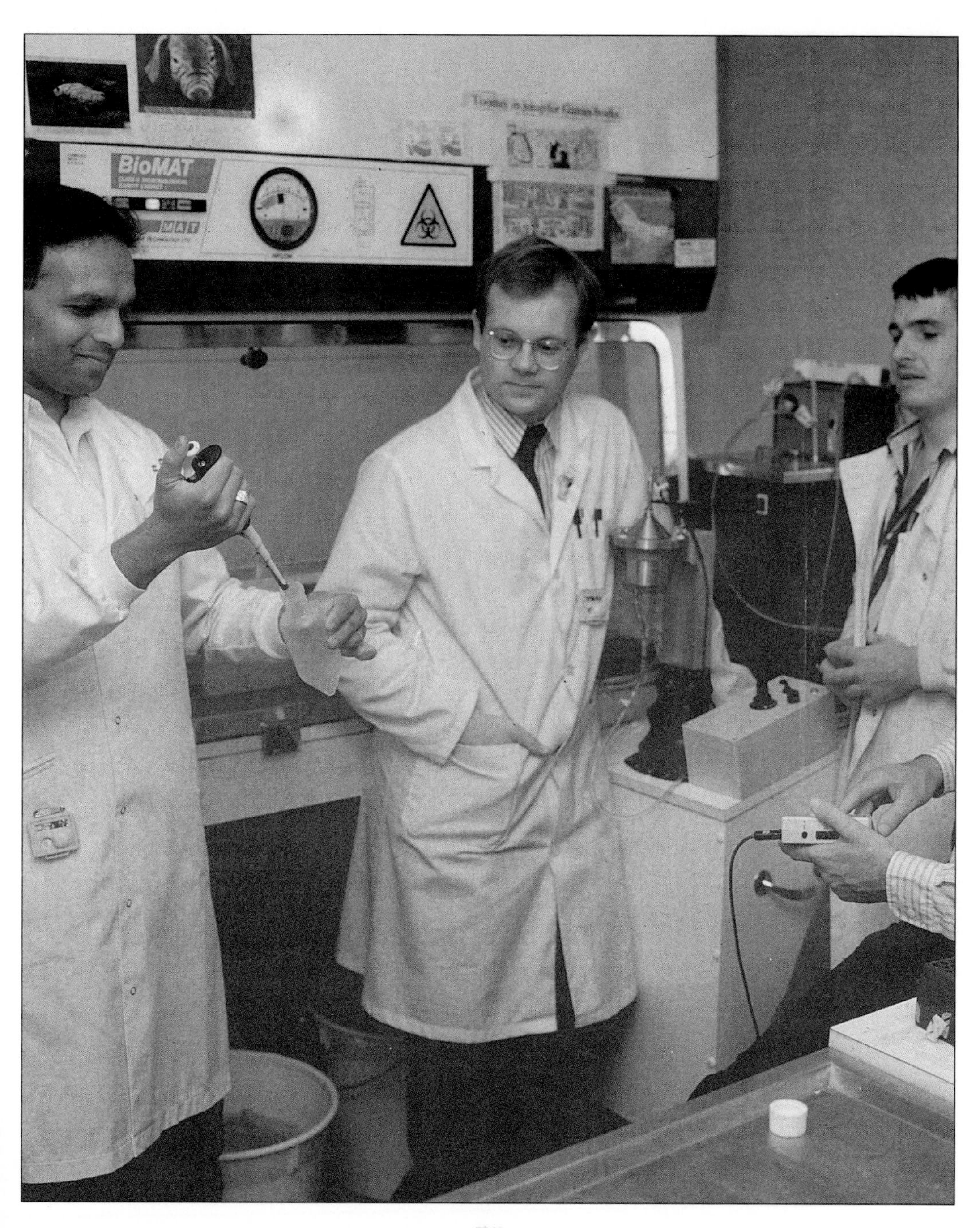
BioMAT

Looking to the future

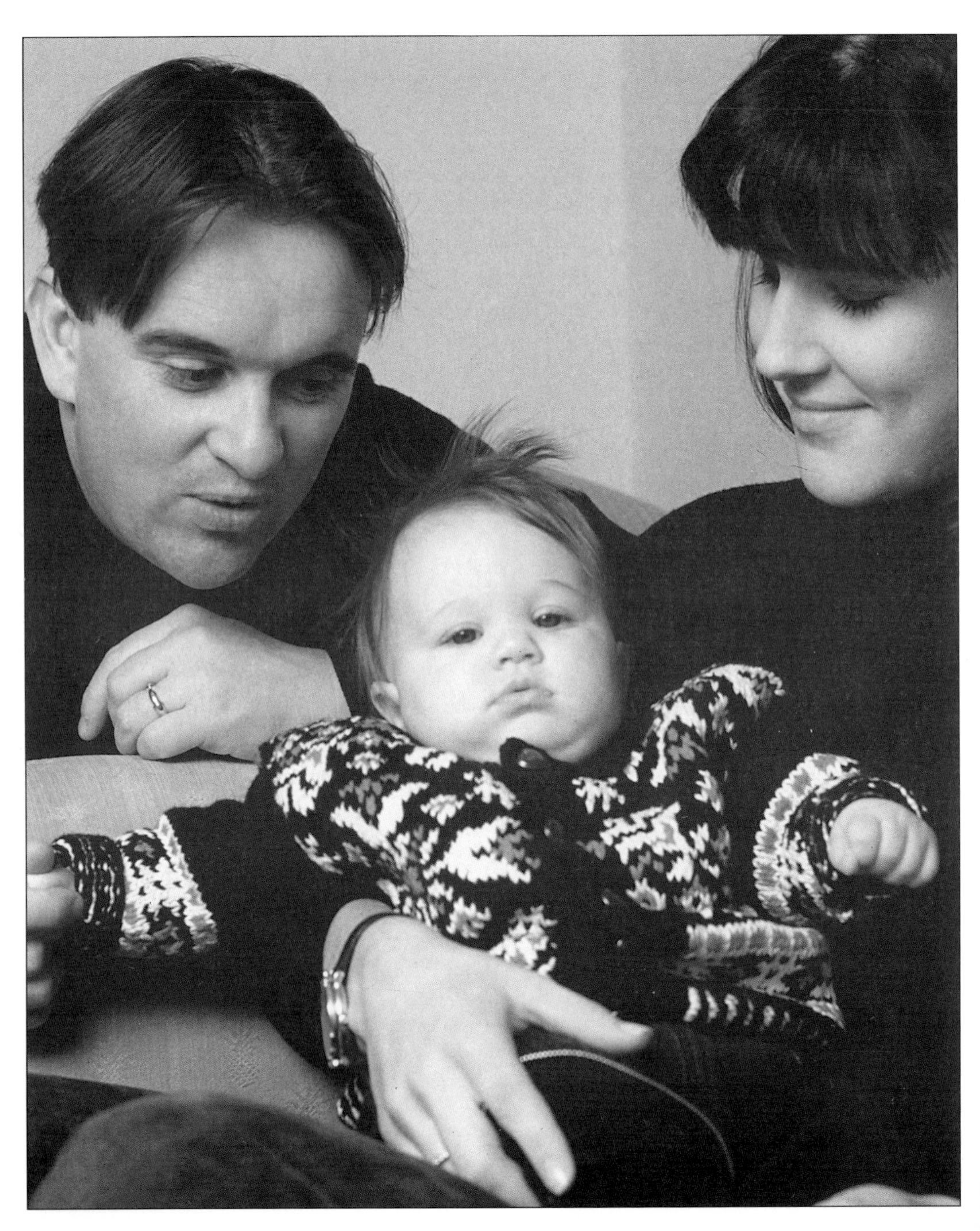

to me to be unlikely."

He believes, however, that research into foetal development may possibly yield interesting findings on diabetes. Certain factors which affect the way a baby develops in the womb could influence whether the individual has the potential to develop diabetes.

One of the areas of greatest optimism is in the prevention of complications. "Blindness caused by retinopathy is now within our control, for example," says Professor Keen. "Regular tests and laser treatment can prevent it, but we need to find ways of picking up those people who may be suffering sight damage because their NIDDMM has not been diagnosed."

It is recognised that some people with diabetes are more likely to develop kidney disease and heart disease, and work is going on to develop an effective screening system which will identify those people at risk at an early stage. Treatment can then be given to slow down, stop or even reverse the development of these conditions before they become serious.

At one time, transplant surgery – to replace either the pancreas itself or the 'islets' which produce insulin – seemed promising, but progress has been slow and many problems remain to be solved. Some work is still going on trying to produce an 'artificial' pancreas, but Professor Keen thinks that success is at least 30 years away.

Interestingly, Professor Keen believes that the greatest advances in the successful management of diabetes have come not in the area of technology but of human care. "The diabetes specialist nurse is the greatest invention since insulin as far as diabetes is concerned," he believes. "Team work is a reality in the sphere of diabetes care and the patient is one of the most important members of that team. The patient's greater understanding of their own diabetes is the single most important factor in living with it successfully and that in itself has transformed the outlook for people with diabetes."

Emergency action for hypoglycaemia

A hypo may occur if an insulin-dependent diabetic has:

1 Eaten insufficient food.
2 Taken too much insulin.
3 Performed strenuous exercise without taking the necessary precautions.

Most diabetics carry an identity card or wear a special engraved bracelet or pendant, which will help the person administering first aid to recognise their condition. They may also carry insulin or some sugar lumps.

Emergency action

1 If the person is conscious, help him to sit down, or lie down, and give him a sweet drink or two sugar cubes. It may help if the sugar cubes are given in water.
2 If the person is semi-conscious or being obstinate and not co-operating, you could smear a little honey or sugar syrup around his mouth.
3 If he is unconscious you must not attempt to give him anything by mouth. Check that his airway is open and that he is breathing and turn him into the recovery position. Seek medical help immediately.

Important

If there is no improvement in the patient's condition within five minutes of giving him sugar, you should seek medical help at once.

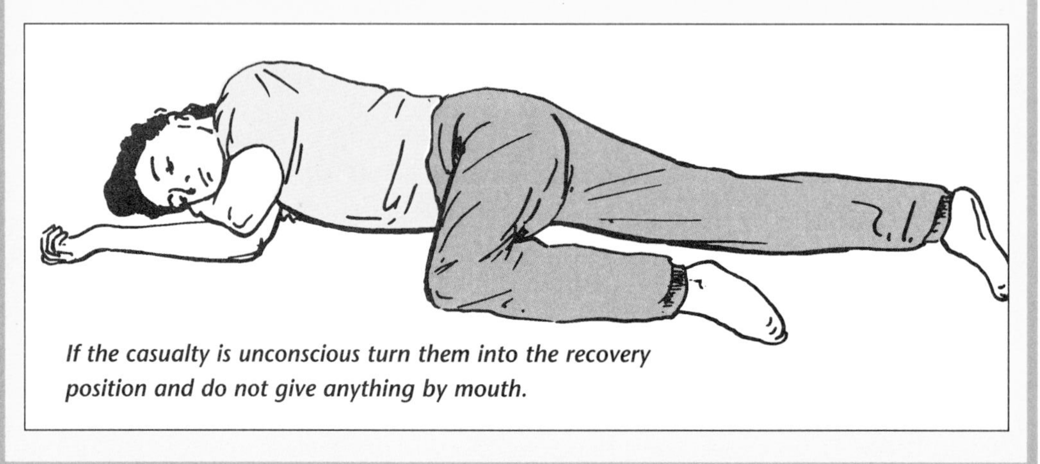

If the casualty is unconscious turn them into the recovery position and do not give anything by mouth.

Useful information

The British Diabetic Association (BDA)
Joining the BDA is one of the most valuable steps that you can take to improve your knowledge about diabetes and get advice and answers to any questions you may have. You can contact the BDA at:
10 Queen Anne Street
London W1M 0BD
Tel: 071 323 1531

Medic-Alert Foundation
This charity sells identity jewellery giving details of the wearer's medical condition. Contact them at:
17 Bridge Wharf
156 Caledonian Road
London N1 9UU
Tel: 071 833 3034

SOS Talisman
This company has a range of jewellery giving all the relevant details of the wearer's medical condition on a folding slip of non-soluble paper.
21 Gray's Corner
Ley Street
Ilford
Essex
Tel: 081 554 5579

Overseas organisations

Australia
Diabetes Australia
QBE Building
33-35 Ainslie Avenue
Canberra A C T
Australia
Tel: 61-62/475655

Canada
Canadian Diabetes Association
78 Bond Street
Toronto
Ontario M5B2J8
Canada
Tel: 1-416/362-4400

New Zealand
Diabetes New Zealand Inc.
4 Coquet Street
PO Box 54
Oamaru
South Island
Tel: 64-3/434 8100

United States
American Diabetes Association
1660 Duke Street
Alexandria
VA 22314
USA
Tel: 1-703/549-1500

Index